Therapy for Stroke
Building on Experience

Margaret Johnstone FCSP

CHURCHILL LIVINGSTONE

EDINBURGH LONDON MELBOURNE NEW YORK AND TOKYO 1991

CHURCHILL LIVINGSTONE
Medical Division of Longman Group UK Limited

Distributed in the United States of America by Churchill
Livingstone Inc., 1560 Broadway, New York, N.Y. 10036,
and by associated companies, branches and representatives
throughout the world.

First published 1991

ISBN 0-443-04625-5

British Library Cataloguing in Publication Data
A catalogue record for this book is available from the British
Library.

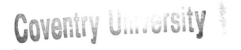
Produced by Longman Singapore Publishers Pte Ltd
Printed in Singapore

Preface

Having travelled extensively in recent years in response to requests to present teaching seminars on stroke rehabilitation, certain questions turn up repeatedly at the question and discussion sessions. This has shown me the need to add one more book to the three I have written previously on stroke rehabilitation. I revised these three books in 1987 but still it seems there is a need to answer some outstanding questions. These answers are presented here.

In the meantime I have continued my own studies in the clinical field. I am greatly indebted to Mrs Ann Thorp, my sister and fellow physiotherapist, who has travelled with me and turned our teaching courses into very successful joint presentations. I also gratefully acknowledge the deeper understanding I have gathered from lectures I have attended given by neurological teachers, in particular Dr M. Hulliger of Zurich, Professor Dr H.-R. Luscher of Bern, Professor Simon Miller of Newcastle and Professor Dr H.P. Clamann of Bern.

I would also like to mention with particular thanks the help and support given to me by Miss Rosemary Lane FCSP, formerly Principal of the Aberdeen School of Physiotherapy, and her invaluable teaching on tonal balance and reflex activity which led to my greater understanding of the stroke patient's rehabilitation needs.

I am also grateful to all the patients who have contributed to my understanding and have so cheerfully cooperated with me in the clinical field.

I would also like to acknowledge the support given to Dr Selz-Keller and myself by Gail Cox Steck, the dedicated physiotherapist who has cheerfully given the leadership and long hours of work that have been necessary over recent years for the successful development and continuing excellence of the neurological rehabilitation unit at Solothurn.

Finally I would like to say how delighted I am that occupational therapists are now attending and working with us on combined teaching seminars. It is essential that we work together for the greater good of the patient. This book is not an update on physiotherapy but rather, as the title suggests, it is a book for the greater cooperation and understanding of all therapists involved in stroke care.

I am greatly indebted to Mary Emmerson Law and Graham Birnie of Churchill Livingstone for their invaluable help in putting this book together.

For the sake of clarity, throughout the text, the patient is referred to as 'he' and the therapist as 'she'.

Edinburgh 1991   Margaret Johnstone

Contents

ERRATUM

Page 60   Line 38
for 'years' read 'months'

1. Neurological background

THE FACTS

This book is intended to present a clear, logical picture of the known facts relating to the neurological damage that may occur in loss of movement due to brain damage from a stroke.

It is impossible to consider or undertake useful rehabilitation of any stroke patient without considering and understanding the possible brain damage that may have taken place. There are a few, already proven, neurological facts that are involved and the consideration of these leads both to the understanding of the disruption of normal movement that may occur, and to ways and means of establishing effective treatment in the clinical field. Hopefully, this points to a way ahead for rehabilitation which can be both useful and effective.

Where reflexes are no longer integrated into cortical control, as in a stroke patient, normal movement is not possible. It is therefore necessary to study the normal in order to assess the abnormal. In this way it becomes possible to plan a useful rehabilitation programme based on impaired movement rather than the normal. All too often therapists have tended to base treatment programmes on the normal or undamaged brain.

It is unrealistic to consider stroke rehabilitation without first understanding the mechanisms involved in the maintenance of *normal muscle tone*. This is because normal movement depends on normal muscle tone and in any disability caused by brain damage due to a stroke, muscle tone is no longer normal. In other words, the therapist should consider the normal to find out if the points relating to normal tone will help towards solving the problems found with abnormal tone. The relevant points to note are that:

1. Normal muscle is balanced.
2. It is reflex in character, based on the reflex arc.
3. It is more marked in the antigravity muscles.

Let us consider these three points one at a time.

1. Normal muscle tone is balanced

For our purpose this fact does not need complicated neurological explanation. Simply consider the normal relationship between the extensors and flexors of the elbow joint. It is useful here to consider the elbow in preference to any other joint because, in stroke rehabilitation, a return to normal movement of the elbow often poses one of the most difficult problems to be overcome. Later a discussion of these difficulties will be presented. The muscles concerned are the *Triceps* and *Biceps*, reciprocally acting muscles, agonists and antagonists.

To extend the elbow the Triceps must contract and, as it contracts, the Biceps must relax if the elbow joint is to extend. So far so good, but why does this reciprocal innervation not occur after the brain damage of stroke? This takes us on to point two.

2. Normal muscle tone is reflex in character, based on the reflex arc

The reflex arc is the basic functional unit of the nervous system. Again neurologists have made this easy for us to understand. As already stated under point one, to extend the elbow the Triceps must contract and, as it contracts, the Biceps must relax. A signal from the brain activates motoneurones in the spinal cord (Fig. 1), the Triceps contracts and the elbow extends. But this cannot happen however unless the Biceps lengthens, or stretches, and this stretch is picked up by stretch receptors which in their turn activate motoneurones in the spinal cord for the Biceps. Thus the Biceps also contracts to resist this stretch and oppose the contraction of the Triceps. This is known as the stretch reflex which, in normal muscle tone, acts to maintain body posture and opposing movement. To be able to extend the elbow this stretch reflex relayed to the Biceps has to be inhibited if normal movement is to occur. This leads us to the conclusion that there has to be some form of inhibition between reciprocally acting muscles.

Inhibitory interneurones in the spinal cord play a crucial role in sequential movement. Study Figure 1 again and note the inhibitory interneurone between the Triceps motoneurone and the Biceps motoneurone and note that this inhibitory motoneurone also receives descending inputs from the brain via the corticospinal tract. Stroke damage takes place in the brain, not in the spinal cord, so any upset in the normal maintenance of balanced muscle tone must come from the brain. It is reasonable and logical therefore to suggest that in the stroke patient this reciprocal inhibition, or balance of muscle tone, has been disrupted by damage to the brain. When considering post-stroke disability, after careful clinical assessment of many patients it seems that the Biceps is continuously contracting making movement very difficult—if not impossible. In recent years leading neurologists

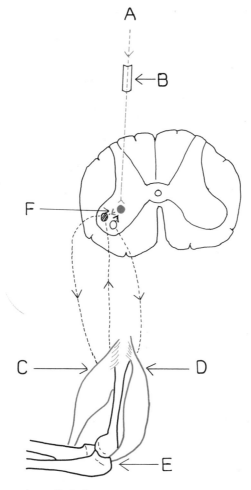

A = Brain input.
B = Corticospinal tracts.
C = Biceps muscle.
D = Triceps muscle.
E = Elbow joint.
F = Inhibitory interneurone.

Fig. 1

have been able to measure the electrical activity of muscles and have demonstrated that post-stroke excitation of antagonist antigravity muscles becomes continuous where spasticity becomes a problem. Here, excitation of the Biceps has become continuous and so, with the stretch reflex in this case no longer under inhibitory control, normal movement about the elbow joint is no longer possible. Presented with such facts, can the rehabilitation therapist find satisfactory answers to the problems presented?

Let us turn to point three.

3. Normal muscle tone is more marked in the antigravity muscles

This being the case, and with the opposing muscle groups out of balance because of lost inhibition from the brain to the stretch reflex, the consequent loss of the necessary reciprocal inhibition will result in severe residual problems.

For many years problem solving of this kind has been left to the physiotherapist. A possible answer can only be found if a satisfactory way of inhibiting the strong antigravity muscles can be introduced. This inhibition would of necessity have to be offered by the environment, by external forces outside the body, by some force for example, which could control and correct the patient's imbalance of muscle tone while rehabilitation is undertaken and reflex activity once more restored to cortical control. Can the therapist really make an effective contribution towards solving the problem?

For many years an attempt has been made to do this by using inhibiting movement patterns and by lying, sitting and standing using inhibiting positioning at all times. But, although this line of thought and specialized treatment makes very sound sense, when offered, it usually comes as too little and too late. Nor can one patient and one therapist go it alone! In many cases strong antigravity patterns have taken over and the patient has become a helpless prisoner held fast in the crippling patterns of spasticity with no chance of regaining normal movement. The urgent need is to start the treatment early after the onset of the stroke and to inhibit 24 hours a day, otherwise we might wonder if there is any point in bothering to treat at all?

For the stroke patient to attain optimum recovery it becomes increasingly obvious that successful exercise programmes must concentrate on control of muscle tone and *control of tonal flow* throughout the whole body while a reasoned and advancing progress scheme is undertaken. All disciplines, physiotherapists, occupational therapists, speech therapists, nurses and doctors should understand the neurological needs of the patient and the reasoning behind this need for meticulous positioning in all treatment sessions and *between treatment sessions*.

And, as if this seemingly difficult task is not enough, there are other problems. Normal movement depends on close interaction between sensory and motor events and, almost always, with our stroke patients we find we are faced with the problems presented by sensory loss. So, more and more it seems like a no win situation and patients and their caring back-up team, be this hospital or home based, become increasingly depressed with the lack of rehabilitation recovery.

SENSORIMOTOR PROBLEMS

The brain receives information through a number of different sensory channels (pathways) and this information is analysed by the Central Nervous System. Previous experience (memory) puts this information into context, it is processed in the brain, which then responds making behaviour immediately appropriate for any environmental situation with the necessary motor responses. Sensorimotor integration is vital if the appropriate responses are to be made to achieve normal movement with postural adjustments as required. Sensorimotor systems have to initiate and coordinate all required movements for any situation and so we understand that the control of movement and posture is dependent on a continuous flow of sensory information about events in the environment. Consider, for example, loss of sensory information about events in systems such as proprioception, vision, hearing and so on. This is one point which some therapists do *not* consider and yet it is of the utmost importance if successful rehabilitation is to be the outcome. The loss of the memory of normal movement probably occurs very quickly after brain damage from stroke and, if the brain is allowed to accept the abnormal and often bizarre movements produced by the released reflexes, it soon becomes a very difficult task to replace the memory of normal movement.

To concentrate on one of the serious post-stroke failures in the sensory systems it is useful, particularly from the physiotherapist's point of view, to study proprioception and the results where loss of proprioception is isolated. Proprioceptive sense is the sense of muscular position or of muscle and joint position. When all the necessary information from proprioceptors is not reaching the sensory cortex due to brain damage, loss of proprioceptive sense will present a serious barrier to any effective rehabilitation. Loss of proprioceptive sense may lead to disturbance of body image—body image being the ability to feel a limb, to appreciate its place in space and its relationship to the body. Tactile sensation may be impaired, or lack of coordination of sensory input may give disturbance of spatial relationships—relationships of objects outside the body. It must be a demoralizing or totally devastating experience for a patient who is no longer aware of his body image and incapable of determining his position in space. Visual agnosia must also be recognised, but as a perceptual problem and not as blindness.*

When considering proprioceptors which are situated in muscles, tendons and joints, and their role in sensory integration, it is also necessary to

---

* Assessment in the whole area of sensory loss is adequately presented in *Restoration of Motor Function in the Stroke Patient*, Margaret Johnstone, Churchill Livingstone, 1987, Third Edition.

consider the role of specialised proprioceptors which lie at musculo-tendinous junctions. These are the Golgi tendon organs; they are receptive to sustained stretch and are known to have an inhibitory influence on motoneurone pools of their own muscle supply—an autogenic effect. Any reaction to sustained stretch of hypertonic muscles should be considered when attempting to restore reciprocal inhibition. The inhibitory influence exerted by the group Ib Golgi tendon organs cannot be ignored. So the question arises, is there a place for sustained stretch in the treatment of stroke and, if so, how may this be applied to the patient?

It is also necessary to consider associated reactions which are very much involved in the rehabilitation of the stroke patient. Associated reactions play a large part in the often all too rapid onset of spasticity in the weeks following a stroke and this, in turn, leads to a serious build-up of residual disabilities. Associated reactions are released postural reactions deprived of voluntary control because of cortical damage. They occur with all attempted movements to give a widespread increase of spasticity and this leads to another question to which the physiotherapist is expected to find an answer, namely, is there an effective way to divert these wayward reactions into inhibiting patterns? Or is the use of inhibiting positioning enough or does it need some form of more dynamic treatment?

Strokes usually result from cerebral thrombosis or haemorrhage and most usually start with an initial stage of hypotonicity, or flaccidity, which all too quickly develops into increasing hypertonicity, or spasticity. But this is not always so and the physiotherapist may be faced with the difficult task of rehabilitating flaccid limbs. Contributing factors to hypotonicity may be associated with cerebral shock, defective afferent information and sensory interruption and, with careful assessment in the clinical field over many years, it was frequently found in cases where proprioceptive sense was deficient.

Again, for many years, it has been the physiotherapist who has been left to find answers to the difficult problems arising because of prolonged hypotonicity and she has not always been able to do this. It has to be remembered that it is not a peripheral problem but a problem of the central nervous system arising from brain damage of the stroke which affects normal function at spinal cord level.

Where sensory interpretation is deficient there is a wide range of assessment tests that may be used to uncover the area of hidden mental damage. Deficit may be found in one or more areas, for example, in intellect, proprioception, communication, perception and so on, and difficulties are often hidden and will cause the patient great mental distress. For instance, physiotherapists and occupational therapists may not be aware of some of the hidden difficulties in communication and here the skilled speech therapist is very much needed. It is a relatively easy task to see the patterns of spasticity and, with hands on the patient, to assess his tonal state and tonal flow. But sensory deficit cannot be seen or felt by the therapist. All therapists should be able to carry out thorough assessment tests and should be able to interpret the test results accurately. There are other proven neurological facts which are logical and have a bearing on the logical and reasonable planning of a sound rehabilitation programme.

For instance, the postural reflex mechanism depends on:

1. Normal postural tone.
2. Normal reciprocal innervation.
3. Normal patterns of movement.

From what has already been said it would seem obvious that the need to rebuild, rehabilitate or restore a normal postural reflex mechanism must be of first importance; therapists must see the need to restore normal postural tone. The difficulty lies in how to set out to do this and, at the same time, to take adequate measures to deal with attendant motor problems such as control of associated reactions. It would also be useful if, at the same time, dynamic sensory input could be offered. Another simple neurological rule states that: 'With dysfunction of the postural reflex mechanism, and where dominant reflexes are no longer under cortical control, spasticity will develop.' Each neurological fact seems to present therapists with more and more rehabilitation problems which may be the outcome from the neurological damage to the brain resulting from a cerebrovascular accident. The therapist's clear aim is to give back to the brain damaged patient *inhibitory control over abnormal patterns of movement*. The purpose is to *restore postural control*. The vestibular system must also be studied as this system is closely concerned with the postural control of muscle tone in relation to gravitational forces. However, stop for a moment and consider! Is there any real need to go more deeply into neurology, or are there enough facts so far on which to base a realistic recovery programme?

The student of neurology may be in danger of becoming too deeply involved in his subject and of finding himself trapped in a vicious circle from which he can see no way out *if* he cannot apply his neurological knowledge to patient treatment. But, by taking the basic and proven neurological rules one at a time, and building on these facts, a relatively simple rehabilitation pattern emerges which frequently leads to highly satisfactory results.

Motor mechanisms are intimately related to, and functionally dependent on, sensory information. Also, the central nervous system can directly control the sensitivity of muscle spindles and the tonic stretch reflex provides the muscle tone necessary for posture. We have already described the stretch reflex and its importance in reciprocal inhibition. Now, take for example, loss of proprioceptive sense where Golgi tendon organs no longer provide information about the tension of muscles, the stretch reflex is affected with resulting abnormal tone. So, with the missing inhibitory input from the brain which has also been described above, add to this a disruption in the necessary sensory information to the brain and the stroke patient is in serious trouble.

These problems are outlined in Figure 2, which represents the major barriers to successful stroke rehabilitation, and a way round these problems has to be found. The question is, what can be done if there is to be any chance of successful rehabilitation?

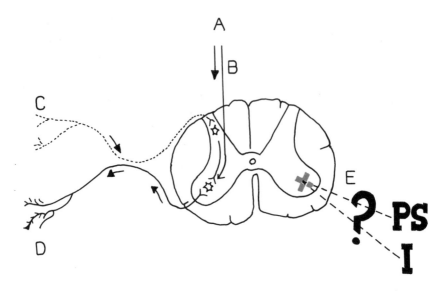

A = Brain input.
B = Corticospinal tracts.
C = Proprioceptors.
D = Muscle spindle.
E = Anterior horn.
PS = Loss of Proprioceptive sense.
I   = Inhibition.

Fig. 2 Major barriers to successful stroke rehabilitation.

2. Apply your neurology

It is helpful to study the facts concerning normal movement as presented in Chapter 1 and to consider the measures that must be taken to make it possible to plan a hopeful physical rehabilitation programme which has a reasonable chance of overcoming the brain damage of stroke. Such a programme should not be stereotyped; it is difficult to find two patients who present in exactly the same way; the physiotherapist should carefully assess each patient and the rehabilitation programme must be based on the findings. But if there is to be reasonable hope of establishing an ongoing recovery programme the basic neurological facts must be understood and effective measures taken to overcome the problems that are found. Let us reconsider the three points made concerning muscle tone.

1. Normal muscle is balanced

In brain damage of stroke, muscle tone is no longer balanced. The reciprocal innovation between agonists and antagonists necessary for normal movement has been disrupted and it is necessary to understand why this has happened in order to shed light on a possible solution to the problem this presents. Is it possible, for example, to restore the balance produced by reciprocal innovation?

2. Normal muscle tone is reflex in character, based on the reflex arc

This point immediately sheds light on a difficult problem and indicates a possible way ahead. The stretch reflex is the key to the problem. In the example given in Chapter 1, to extend the elbow the stronger antagonist (Biceps) must relax to allow the movement to take place, but as soon as the agonist (Triceps) starts to act by initiating the movement of extension, the stretch reflex tells the Biceps to contract. In normal movement the built-in inhibition between reciprocally acting muscles inhibits the stretch reflex to the Biceps and allows extension to take place. Normal movement depends on normal muscle tone. Normal muscle tone is reflex in character, based on the reflex arc. So, an upset in reciprocal innervation clearly implies that the stroke has caused brain damage. Neurologists have aided our understanding of what happens by scientific tests which measure the electrical activity of the muscles and demonstrate that post-stroke excitation of antagonist antigravity muscles becomes continuous where spasticity becomes a problem. In extension of the elbow the Biceps is the antigravity muscle which is affected, disrupting normal movement. The problem for therapists is whether they can find a method of treatment that will compensate or provide a substitute for the missing tonal balance. In other words, is it possible to do for the patient what his brain can no longer do? Is there some effective way of supplying the missing inhibition—because that is what is necessary?

3. Normal muscle tone is more marked in the antigravity muscles

Obviously, where normal muscle tone has been more marked pre-stroke, post-stroke, with the missing inhibitory input from the brain, this must present an enormous problem and this problem *must* be faced and an effective method of dealing with it must be found. So, this missing inhibitory input must now be offered by some outside influence, some influence which could effectively control and correct the patient's imbalance of muscle tone while rehabilitation is undertaken. And this is not simply to consider movement of one joint (as in the elbow). Consideration must immediately be given to the whole body and to complete patterns of movement throughout the whole body. Those who set out on the difficult task of presenting a hopeful and effective rehabilitation programme are faced with the problem of restoring movement patterns other than those produced by reflexes which are no longer under cortical control. Can therapists really be expected to offer an effective way of dealing with this enormous problem?

For many years the answer to the problem has been accepted as the need to *use inhibitory positioning*. Positioning means the use of positions which oppose the strong antigravity patterns. The patient must be nursed in these corrective positions and must be handled using patterns of movement opposed to the antigravity patterns. So, corrective inhibiting positioning must be based on a study of these strong antigravity patterns before inhibitory patterns will be clearly understood. Positioning should also take into account the influence exerted on the distribution of muscle tone where the patient is lying, sitting or standing (see Fig. 3). For example, in lying the stroke patient is frequently placed, or allowed to be, on his back. But lying on the back is the position of greatest extensor tone, whilst lying on the side is the most neutral position. To hold the body upright in a standing position, the whole body is using a total extension pattern against gravity

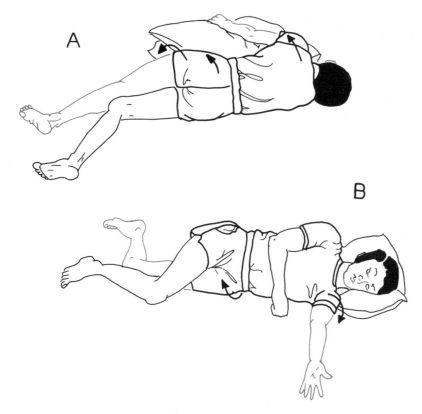

Fig. 3 Inhibitory patterns: A = Lying on the sound side; B = Lying on the affected side.

except for the elbow, wrist and fingers where the antigravity pattern is flexion. This must mean that *inhibiting* patterns for the whole body will be flexion patterns except for the forearm and hand where the inhibiting pattern is extension. (This gives us the most important single influence concerned in failure of rehabilitation of the stroke disabled arm.) Nurses who are not taught these simple facts can hardly be expected to be efficient members of any rehabilitation team. And, if an inhibitory influence is to be offered 24 hours a day, it is nurses who are usually with the patient round the clock and therefore have a very important part to play.* It cannot make

---

* *The Stroke Patient—A Team Approach*, Margaret Johnstone, Churchill Livingstone, 1987, Third Edition, and *Home Care for the Stroke Patient*, Margaret Johnstone, Churchill Livingstone, 1987, Second Edition.

sense to allow the patient to lie stretched out on his back. One night of lying on his back can destroy any advance in rehabilitation that has been made during the day. Or, if the patient is cared for at home and the caring family member is not taught corrective positioning, rehabilitation progress will be diminished.

The rehabilitation programme aims at restoring the postural reflex mechanism, and, therefore, at restoring postural tone, leading to normal reciprocal innervation and normal patterns of movement. It is helpful to have guidelines on which to base a positive and dynamic progress plan. For example:

1. Make a sound and positive decision about which muscles must be considered as the main antigravity supports.
2. Decide where and how to make a start.
3. Look at total tonal patterns and consider associated reactions.
4. Consider ways and means of introducing inhibitory practice.
5. What does the programme offer where there is marked proprioceptive loss?

Considered in this way there is a logical and practical course to be followed.

1. Make a sound and positive decision about which muscles must be considered as the main antigravity muscles

The chief muscles by which the erect posture is maintained will be closely involved in extension of the trunk which will include trunk to shoulder and trunk to hip. For this gross motor pattern there are two main muscles to consider:

(i) *Latissimus dorsi*: which is a large triangular-shaped muscle which has its origin in the posterior part of the iliac crest and the spinous processes of the lumbar and lower thoracic vertebrae. It passes obliquely upwards across the back and under the arm to be inserted by a narrow tendon into the floor of the bicipital groove of the humerus (hence the shoulder involvement). It is the broadest muscle of the back. With its extensive origins it covers a large area of the trunk and assists in extension which involves the shoulder joint. It also extends, retracts and *inwardly rotates* the shoulder, drawing the arm downwards and backwards.

(ii) *Gluteus maximus*: which forms the main bulk of the buttock. It originates from the outer surface of the iliac bone and the sacrum and is inserted into the upper end of the femur. It is the muscle chiefly concerned with the maintenance of the erect posture and this explains why it is much more developed in man than in animals. It extends, retracts and *outwardly rotates* the hip.

2. Decide where and how to make a start

The spasticity pattern in the trunk area will lead to an immobile scapula with trunk shortening and side flexion to the affected side and extension, retraction and *inward rotation* of the shoulder. In the lower trunk it will lead to a similar problem in the hip with hip extension, retraction and—this time—*outward rotation*. In other words these spasticity patterns are set by the uninhibited actions of *Latissimus dorsi* and *Gluteus maximus* because the inhibitory input from the brain is missing. Reciprocal innervation is lacking. So, start with the trunk and decide how to take action to avoid developing spasticity. Careful positioning *must* be included in the rehabilitation pro-gramme to prevent excessive development of antigravity tone which would lead to lateral shortening of the trunk and severe shoulder problems. Likewise, developing spasticity of the hip must be inhibited by positioning in the pattern which opposes the action of *Gluteus maximus*.

Stroke disability is all too often thought of as loss of normal movement in the arm and the leg. But, with the large trunk origins of the chief muscles which maintain man's erect posture, we cannot afford to neglect the dis-ability which occurs in the trunk.

3. Look at total tonal patterns and consider associated reactions

As long as it is possible to find in any 'caring' situation a stroke patient who has been instructed to struggle hard to perform a task with a disabled hand while the rest of the arm is held fast in increasing spasticity we must recognise that there is still a great need in all branches of the medical world for more education in respect of brain damage to be found after a cere-brovascular accident. Such practices cannot result in normal function of the hand; indeed, in such a case, the patient is being encouraged to increase his disability. There is a great and urgent need for better understanding of the neurological result where:

a. The inhibitory input from the brain no longer has any influence on the maintenance of normal muscle tone.

b. Also, and equally important, there is a great need for full understand-ing of total tonal patterns. This understanding must include normal pat-terns as well as the abnormal patterns resulting from the lack of inhibitory control and, therefore, the lack of reciprocal innervation.

4. Consider ways and means of introducing inhibitory practice

First return to the shoulder joint and remember that the extensive and very strong antigravity muscle *Latissimus dorsi* is now in a state where the stretch reflex is no longer inhibited and, with release from cortical control, spas-ticity will develop. This sets the spasticity pattern for the shoulder. But, this is not the whole picture. Any movement (and this movement also includes the sound side of the body, that is, the total body) will give overflow of tone all down the affected side of the patient. Again, taking the arm as an illustration, this overflow of muscle tone will spread down the arm and will follow a course set by the stronger antigravity muscles of the forearm. This means that the forearm and hand will very soon build up excessive and unwanted tone in the flexors of the forearm and hand—and this spasticity pattern also usually includes pronation.

Remembering the definition of associated reactions leads to understanding the urgent need to know the antigravity patterns. Associated reactions are released postural reactions deprived of voluntary control because of cortical damage. They occur with all attempted movements to give a widespread increase of spasticity. So, where arm spasticity is involved, the more a patient struggles to use a disabled hand the quicker excessive spasticity will develop. We may also come across a ludicrous situation where a test for hand disability is presented as taking up the handshake grasp with the patient and then asking him to 'squeeze my hand'. This involves flexing the fingers as strongly as possible (the total spasticity pattern). If such a test is to make any sense at all the command ought to be to 'let go of my hand'. The tester will then be able to feel any ability there may be to leave the flexion pattern of spasticity and make an active movement into the antigravity pattern of extension.

The arm has been used to illustrate the total spasticity pattern of the upper limb because, judging by the poor rehabilitation results, it seems that it is particularly difficult to recover full function of the hemiplegic arm. But this is again readily understood as soon as tonal patterns, both normal and abnormal, are understood. They must be seen as total patterns and not simply as the patterns of isolated and separate joints. The total spasticity pattern for the arm begins in the upper trunk and spreads to include extension with inward rotation of the shoulder and flexion of the elbow, wrist and fingers, usually with pronation of the forearm. In this case it is the strong antigravity pattern of *Latissimus dorsi* which leads on into the total spasticity pattern of the arm. It is vital to inhibit this from *Day 1 of the onset of the stroke*. Unless the therapist is able to visualise this in her mind's eye, and also to visualise the total opposing pattern which will give the necessary inhibition to developing spasticity, she is unlikely to be able to offer satisfactory rehabilitation measures.

It has been suggested that rehabilitation should begin with the trunk but, if this approach is to lead towards a successful treatment plan, we now see a very urgent need to hold the arm in the inhibiting pattern to control tonal flow while the trunk is mobilised. It is not possible to rehabilitate an arm on an unstable trunk; also it is necessary to give the arm stability in the corrective pattern while work on the trunk goes ahead to produce trunk stability.

An amusing illustration of the problem is represented in Figure 4 but it is not, however, an amusing situation for the patient. Compare the whole working wheel with the whole man—the hub of the wheel is the central support. In man this central support is the trunk. But damage to the hub of the wheel will cause collapse of the spokes; damage to the neurological working of the trunk causes the man to collapse. Neither the wheel nor the man can function normally without central stability. A vicious circle one may think, yet it need not be providing a satisfactory way can be found to maintain inhibiting patterns (particularly in the arm), and to allow for early corrective weightbearing while rehabilitation is undertaken. It is essential to follow certain principles which are based on sound neurology. Loss of proprioception will be discussed later.

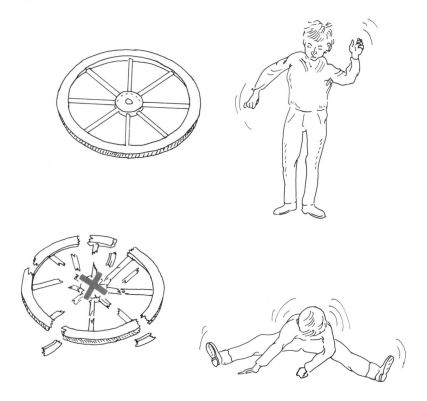

Fig. 4   Start with the trunk.

START WITH THE TRUNK

Working to restore trunk mobility and stability will inevitably, in the early days, include rolling and stabilising techniques and, while this is undertaken, associated reactions must be controlled. For example, rolling over from supine to side-lying is a total flexion pattern. Flexion of the shoulder is the inhibitory pattern, but, for the rest of the arm, this flexion pattern must be diverted into the inhibiting pattern of extension if forearm recovery is to go ahead. This one example of the required inhibitory input which the brain can no longer offer to maintain normal tone illustrates very well the need for some outside inhibitory influence to be offered by the therapist if this missing brain function is to be prevented from permanently destroying postural control. That is, the therapist's clear aim is to give back to the brain damaged patient inhibitory control over abnormal patterns of movement. There are not enough therapists, however, to go round the large number of hemiplegic patients waiting for rehabilitation, nor have individual therapists enough time to spend on individual patients. To give the hemiplegic arm stability in the necessary inhibitory pattern, even should it be found to be possible to do this while working on the trunk, of necessity treatment sessions would be too short to achieve any significant results.

Conclusion. It is relatively easy to control and maintain corrective leg patterns. From the waist downwards inhibiting tonal patterns are flexion patterns. But, from the waist upwards, although inhibiting patterns are flexion patterns up to and including the shoulder, the inhibiting tonal pattern for the elbow, wrist and fingers must be directed into extension. Therein lies the main reason for our frequent failure to recover controlled movement of the hand.

Note. It should be noted that the inhibiting patterns quoted here apply to the majority of hemiplegic patients. In some cases the spasticity patterns (for various reasons which will be discussed later) do not follow the general pattern but each patient *must* be assessed separately and therapists *must treat what they find.*

THE ORALLY INFLATABLE PRESSURE SPLINT

A suitable tool which will greatly assist the maintenance of inhibiting patterns in the hemiplegic arm, controlling tonal flow and giving stability while rehabilitation is undertaken, is found in the orally inflatable pressure splint as illustrated in Figure 5.

This splint, in the form of a double sleeve, is made of specially developed PVC-sheeting, and, with inflation, the space between the double sleeve swells up so that the enclosed limb becomes cushioned with all over even pressure which maintains the limb's position and gives stability. It is usually applied with the patient lying in the total spasticity inhibiting pattern, that

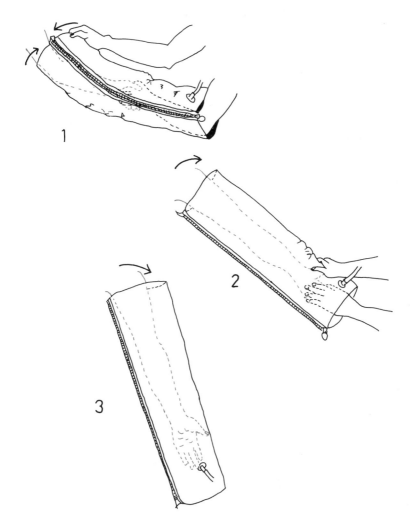

Fig. 5 Application of the long arm splint in three easy stages.

is, with both the patient's knees bent up, maintaining the flexion pattern in the lower half of the body, and with the head extended and rotated towards the affected side with pillow support to maintain neck extension and shoulder flexion with outward rotation. The head position is important neurologically. With neck extension and head rotation to the affected side tonic neck reflexes are assisting tonal correction (inhibition of flexor spasticity) in the elbow, wrist and fingers. The splint is applied as shown in 1, 2 and 3 in Figure 5. Applied in this sequence it illustrates the easiest method to follow to ensure that the arm is in outward rotation with the

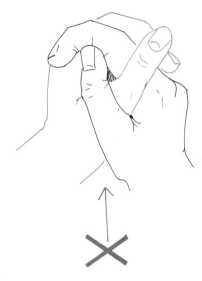

Fig. 6 Use the hand clasped position but palms must be pressed firmly together with elbows extended to maintain outward rotation of the shoulder.

elbow, wrist and fingers extended and the *thumb abducted*. It is also necessary to make sure that the splint is positioned with the fingers well back from the open end and the top of the splint must not press into the axilla. The splint should only be inflated by mouth to ensure that warm, moist air softens and moulds the inner sleeve to conform evenly with the limb; the limb itself being enclosed in a fine cotton sleeve to avoid skin contact with the plastic and prevent a possible sweat reaction. The splint should never be worn in bright sunlight.

The **uses** of the splint will be immediately apparent:

1. The therapist's need for *extra hands* to assist in maintaining the spasticity inhibiting pattern of extension in the forearm and hand is taken over by this splint control.

2. The arm *stability* which is missing but necessary when trunk rehabilitation is undertaken is instantly supplied by splint support. It should be used from the earliest days, for example while mobilising and stabilising the upper trunk and shoulder.

3. All *associated reactions* are diverted away from the antigravity patterns of spasticity.

4. It allows *early weightbearing* to take place through the affected limb while it is maintained in the inhibiting pattern. Weightbearing increases tone: weightbearing through the inhibiting pattern will therefore increase the weak tonal pattern. It is necessary to get corrective tone into the upper trunk and shoulder as quickly as possible if shoulder problems are to be

avoided and so this becomes an essential (and now possible) part of any effective treatment.

5. *Sensory loss*, which must always be considered and sensory input will be given a boost by pressure from the splint. If clasped hands are used as an inhibitory position, note Figure 6.

To return to the **vicious circle** faced in the rehabilitation of the hemiplegic arm and the suggestion that it need not remain a vicious circle provided a satisfactory method is used to maintain inhibiting patterns and to allow early weightbearing, the skilled use of the inflatable pressure splint now presents a way ahead.

Controlling tonal flow

Next it was necessary to consider the question of sustained stretch and its bearing on successful treatment. Obviously the inflatable pressure splint correctly applied to the arm will hold the forearm flexors (the antigravity muscles) in a position of sustained stretch. If the Golgi tendon organs are receptive to sustained stretch and are known to have an inhibitory influence on motoneurones of their own muscle supply—an autogenic effect—a scientific test to prove the worth of the arm splint would be very useful at this stage. Thanks to the help offered to me by Dr Geoffrey Walsh and his research team of the Department of Physiology, University Medical School, Edinburgh, I was able to verify this point. Using a machine which Dr Walsh had himself developed and his department was using to measure muscle tone using printed motors as torque generators we were able to set up a trial to record EMG readings on wrist compliance measurements, testing severe flexor spasticity in a series of hemiplegic arms. Readings were taken *before* pressure splint application and *after* removal of the splint approximately one hour later.[*]

The conclusion of this trial gave a clear and very positive result; tonic and phasic flexor EMG was much reduced and responses had become much more 'plastic' with moulding of the wrist into extension as the flexors yield. Now, some 10 years later, I have still not established the carry over period for this reduction in spasticity. In the clinical field patients frequently report that they 'feel' a marked improvement in the limb, it is not so 'tight', they sleep better, former pain has gone and, from a rehabilitation point of view, in many cases the rate of recovery in hand function has been remarkable. With late treatment, where severe spasticity has already taken over, it is much more difficult to reverse the disability, but, although the success rate

[*]   An example of the readings obtained and a report on the trial is given in the preface of *Restoration of Motor Function in the Stroke Patient*, Margaret Johnstone, Churchill Livingstone, 1987, Third Edition.

is not so high, there have been some very satisfactory results. Treatment based on sound neurological principles should begin early—from the day of onset patients should be positioned in inhibiting patterns and wherever possible they should be taught corrective positioning. Special attention should always be given to the shoulder joint. The unconscious patient is usually turned from one side to the other every 2 hours. If he is rolled over onto a hemiplegic shoulder which is trapped in inward rotation under his body weight severe damage to the shoulder will result; once the agony shoulder syndrome has begun—and, if further poor handling is continued any hope of a successful rehabilitation outcome will be destroyed. No damage will occur where outward rotation with protraction is maintained in this most vulnerable joint.

5. What does the programme offer where there is marked proprioceptive loss?

Applying the full arm splint correctly to maintain the inhibiting pattern of extension in the elbow, wrist and fingers, giving stability and diverting tonal flow into the inhibiting pattern, is only *part* of the treatment. Using the pressure splint must not be purely a *passive* treatment. There is much *active* work which must also be done (while the splint maintains the necessary inhibiting pattern and controls associated reactions) if patients are to reach a high standard of recovery (study Fig. 7). The pressure splint offers a solution to the capital I in Figure 2. With the introduction of this rehabilitation tool in the clinical field it became possible in many cases to restore a working hand with skilled movement. But there remained those who, in spite of early treatment, failed to recover hand function. Making a careful study of assessment findings in a long series of severely disabled stroke patients it became clear that the patients who fitted this category of failure all had marked to severe loss of proprioceptive sense (see PS in Fig. 2).

The advancing exercise programme offered to all the patients in many ways followed the developmental patterns of the infant. Progress went from rolling patterns to crawling patterns, high kneeling led to standing; or in some cases, particularly in the very elderly, progress came through rolling to sitting to standing.

During this advancing progress the levels of reflex activity are taken into account. These levels are **spinal, tonic, basal** and **cortical**. All levels from Spinal upwards can be modified but Basal level is required before Cortical level can be effective. The aim is to get back to Cortical level so that dominant reflexes are once more integrated into Cortical control. Spinal level has already been discussed and a possible way of dealing with the loss of inhibition on the reflex arc has been suggested. Tonic responses will obviously play an important role in rehabilitation, particularly in the early

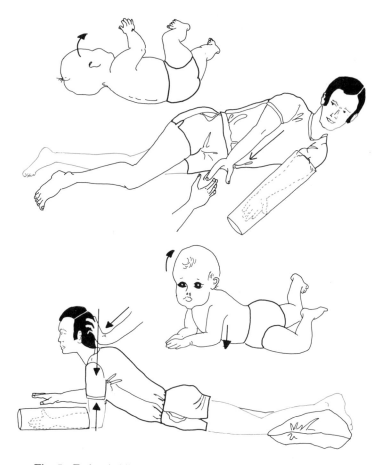

Fig. 7   Early rehabilitation patterns related to motor development.

days. These are the midbrain responses, tonic neck reflexes and labyrin-thine responses. The position of the patient's head is important; neck flexion increases unwanted flexor tone in the forearms but this effect is controlled in exercise when the arm splint is in place.

Early trunk rolling patterns are used from the beginning to establish and maintain trunk mobility and to assist in regaining balance. Tonic responses are stereotyped primitive responses which are modified or overruled at higher levels *when the postural reflex mechanism is fully established.* They produce involuntary changes in muscle tone in response to stimulation of sensory nerve endings, namely, exteroceptors and proprioceptors. Thera-pists involved in stroke rehabilitation should have a sound knowledge of the levels of reflex activity. This is particularly necessary if assessment tests are to give a true picture of the individual patient's stage or state of recovery with a bearing on the planning of the individual rehabilitation programme. For example, rapid rolling will have a profound effect on the position of the patient's head and the inner ear, the vestibular system will give an increased reaction to stretch stimuli and, where necessary if these responses cannot be modified at higher levels as in the brain damage of stroke, development of flexor spasticity in the forearm may be very rapid.

The therapist's two hands are not enough to control inhibiting patterns in the forearm and are needed elsewhere to apply the manual contacts which will meet the necessary rehabilitation needs by assisting or resisting movement patterns and suitably altering tonal flow in any ongoing exercise programme. Exercises in lower trunk rotations will inhibit unwanted extensor tone in the lower half of the body. The more the therapist understands about the development of controlled muscle tone, the more it would seem to make sound sense to follow the development patterns of the infant in stroke rehabilitation *provided* it is possible, at the same time, to supply the necessary inhibitory input. As total inhibitory patterns are flexion patterns **except for the forearm and hand**, use of the long arm pressure splint would seem to make this programme possible.

THE PROBLEM OF SEVERE LOSS OF PROPRIOCEPTIVE SENSE

It had taken 10 years in the clinical field to establish the use of the pressure splint in the prevention of developing spasticity (and I shall always be indebted to Dr Geoffrey Walsh and his research team). It took 5 more years in the clinical field to produce facts and figures which would present and support a useful solution to the problem of severe loss of proprioceptive sense. In the case of motor loss, following neurodevelopmental patterns combined with a satisfactory method of inhibition was giving a high rate of recovery. In the case of sensory loss there now became an urgent need to find a way to further boost sensory input. Various methods had been tried during the first 10 years, such as weightbearing through joints where the splint gave stability in inhibiting patterns to stimulate joint proprioceptors but this had not proved to be adequate. Loss of proprioceptive sense (PS) remained an unsolved problem.

Where assessment had not uncovered sensory loss, and when it became possible to strongly inhibit excessive muscle tone, it had made very good sense to attempt to restore motor function by following the infant's developmental patterns. This was not the case where brain damage of the stroke disturbed sensory interpretation. It now seemed a logical step to consider sensory development and to go even further back to the pre-birth days of the developing fetus. Here developing sensation was influenced by three major inputs: touch, movement and pressure. Pressure splints supplied all three of these necessary inputs but, with the loss of proprioceptive sense, this had not proved enough to achieve satisfactory results. But what was lacking? Failure lay perhaps not in touch and pressure but in altering pressures. As the fetus grows, pressure increases and the pressure constantly varies with the mother's breathing and movements. The safe pressure from the sustained pressure splint had been judged to be no more than the full inflation that could be applied when the splint was blown up by mouth, that is, 40 mmHg. Also it was felt that lung pressure could not overinflate. Later we discovered that a man who played the Highland bagpipe could overinflate. So if in doubt, test with a sphygmomanometer. Also, it should not be forgotten that warm, moist air from the lungs will soften and mould the inner sleeve of the splint to conform with the limb.

It was a logical step to consider the use of intermittent pressure produced by a machine in the search for a solution to the problem presented by proprioceptive loss. Inflation pressure should be no more than 40 mmHg, deflation pressure should drop considerably. Very soon other workers in the field were using intermittent pressure, inflation going as high as 70 mmHg, and were claiming this treatment reduced spasticity. It became urgently necessary to establish the safe and useful pressure that ought to be used. Once again Dr Geoffrey Walsh offered the help of his team and we set up a blood flow trial led by Dr Joan Gelman. Using strain gauge equipment we measured blood flow through hemiplegic arms before and after treatment by intermittent pressure. There are various pumps on the market. We used the British Flowpulse 1100 machine, supplied by Huntleigh Medical Ltd. This machine offers:

Pressure: Variable 20–100 mmHg.
Inflation Time: Variable in steps 3 seconds–4 minutes.
Deflation Time: Variable in steps 3 seconds–4 minutes.
Treatment Time: Variable up to 1 hour.

The conclusion from our study was that pressures alternating from 40 mmHg for 3 seconds to 10 mmHg for 3 seconds were the correct pressures to be given—the 3 second sequence was chosen because that was the shortest time the machine could give. We were attempting to mimic the effect of a mother's breathing and movements on the sensory development of the growing fetus. Our conclusion was based on the fact that higher pressures resulted in hypoxic limbs. That a limb was suffering from a degree of hypoxia was borne out by finding increased blood flow following the release of intermittent pressure where higher pressures up to 70 mmHg were used. It had been shown by other workers that 25 minutes of hypoxia can alter sensation of the four modalities, *touch and pressure* disappearing before *temperature and pain*.

Since hypoxic muscle loses its tone it was not surprising that some therapists had found spasticity had decreased in limbs subjected to the higher alternating pressures which produced hypoxia. We suggested that the use of higher pressures should be discontinued on the grounds that a further loss of sensation might very well occur in some patients and that the decrease in spasticity could only be due to ischaemia of the muscles concerned and therefore a temporary phenomenon. Indeed, with a build-up of subsequent treatments it was found that returning spasticity became steadily more marked. This study led to our statement that this type of mechanical treatment should only be used for our purpose provided carefully correct pressures are given (as stated above).

Next, I collected six patients with severe loss of proprioceptive sense. This did not present a problem as I was working in a long term hospital which admitted patients who had failed to rehabilitate elsewhere. The intermittent pressure regime described above was given twice daily for 45 minutes. The treatment time of 45 minutes was chosen of necessity because this was all that could be fitted into a busy working day and all six patients were also taking part in the full rehabilitation programme using all sustained pressure techniques. All six of these initial trial patients made very satisfactory rehabilitation progress and recovered hand function. It should be noted that although the complete programme takes up considerable time in each working day, by using pressure splints and pressure techniques it is possible for two therapists to treat up to fifteen severely disabled stroke patients adequately in each day.* With plastic bifurcations up to four limbs were treated simultaneously.

I am indebted to Professor George Adams. I used his book *Cerebrovascular Disability and the Ageing Brain* (Churchill Livingstone 1974) in my earlier clinical research days to help me in my attempts to understand the mysteries of sensory loss. In a second study of this book in 1979 I particularly noted one paragraph which stated:

'Defective proprioception denies the patient the assured knowledge of joint position and movement essential to the recovery of mobility. The servo system concerned in antigravity and postural mechanisms is dependent on it, and even when motor power and intellect are well preserved, loss of proprioception *results in severe and persistent handicap*.' (my italics)

It was this statement that set me off on a search to find an answer to this serious problem.

Adding intermittent pressure to the treatment programme seemed to give an answer to the problem of proprioceptive loss. It is important to note that all six patients in the initial trial had previously failed to rehabilitate in our intensive unit offering all sustained pressure techniques. Since then results

---

* *Contra-indications*: This type of mechanical alteration in pressure should not be used on patients in acute pulmonary oedema and should be used with caution on those with congestive heart failure or in those where pre-existing deep venous thrombosis is suspected.

have been very encouraging with only a small percentage of failures. A possible explanation for improved treatment results might be related to sensory development of the fetus and the altering pressures as the mother breathes.

More recently I have used Huntleigh Medical's Flopac machine. It is smaller than their Flowpulse machine and easily portable but does not have a deflation pressure and inflation time will not go lower than 5 seconds. However it appears to be quite satisfactory if it inflates up to 40 mmHg for 5 seconds and simply deflates for 5 seconds. It should be noted that the sleeves supplied with these machines are not transparent. This makes it difficult to establish that the patient's arm *and hand* are fully maintained in the inhibiting pattern. I undertook the study and all subsequent treatments using the URIAS long arm splint. Where a compression boot is used on the lower leg it is easy to position the patient in sitting using the boot supplied with the machine; when the longer full length boot is used special care must be taken to maintain the leg in slight elevation with the hip in inward rotation.

3. The basic concept

The sensorimotor approach is based on the concept that an organism functions by a cycle of sensory input from within and outside the body, being integrated within the brain, where a decision is made about the necessary action. If action is taken then further feedback from sensory end organs confirms whether this has been carried out as required. There will be a continuous monitoring and correction of the response to ensure that the appropriate action is either carried out or maintained. When there is damage to this system lower reflex responses are no longer inhibited by the brain and therefore abnormal responses take place. With disturbance of the finely balanced inhibitory–facilitatory responses, abnormalities of muscle tone and posture occur. The rehabilitation programme aims at primarily controlling tonal and postural patterns so that the patient may obtain optimal benefit from natural neurological recovery. It cannot be overemphasised that rehabilitation is a 24-hour a day process and therefore all members of hospital staff, relatives, helpers and the patient himself must understand what is being attempted and the techniques for achieving these goals.

The neurophysiological aims are:

1. Inhibit dominant reflexes.
2. Facilitate specific responses.
3. Improve postural control.
4. Increase sensory input.
5. Re-establish lost responses.
6. Facilitate cortical control and feedback.

The rehabilitation programme will include:

1. Instituting a round-the-clock programme of corrective positioning to influence the distribution of muscle tone.
2. Using a planned programme of activities which gradually progress

through stages as each level of competence has been achieved. Stability in one stage is achieved before progressing to the next.

3. The programme is based on the motor development patterns of the infant.

4. Weightbearing through correctly placed joints is an important part of the recovery programme.

5. The use of inflatable pressure splints to:

(a) Inhibit dominant reflex patterns.

(b) Give the stability of sustained posture.

(c) Offer prolonged stretch to the sensory receptors in muscles and tendons—by decreasing the sensory feed back, spasticity is decreased.

(d) Inhibit associated reactions.

(e) Assist in early weightbearing through correctly positioned joints.

The advancing rehabilitation programme follows two possible distinct routines:

1. Rolling to sitting to standing to walking.

2. Rolling to prone lying to stabilising propping on elbows to crawling to kneeling to standing to walking.

Note. That whichever routine is followed corrective shoulder and hip patterns must be maintained at all times. The two routines are interchangeable though the first may sometimes be more suitable for the elderly patient who has associated arthritis of back, hips or knees. Prone lying with elbow propping, kneeling and crawling in this situation will cause pain and is therefore to be avoided. Wherever possible the patient should take the responsibility for his own positioning, the therapist or helper gradually withdrawing support.

There are three rules of fundamental importance:

1. *Start early* after onset of the stroke. (Even the unconscious patient must be maintained in corrective positioning of shoulder and hip.)

2. Maintain corrective positioning *at all times.*

3. *Everyone* who has any dealings with the patient must be instructed in corrective positioning. The patient learns to live in the patterns of recovery which are based on inhibiting patterns.

A BROAD OUTLINE OF THE TREATMENT PLAN

It is necessary to understand normal movement.

Normal movement depends on:

1. Normal tone

Must be (a) high enough, and (b) low enough.

2. Normal patterns of movement

Developed from primitive reflex movement present at birth to weightbearing with mobility and skills. Automatic—Voluntary—Selective. True recovery of normal must have automatic movement.

3. Normal postural reflex mechanism

(a) Righting reactions:
    head righting
    rotating within the body axis
(b) Equilibrium reactions:
    moving the body against a fixed support
    moving the support
    protective extension
(c) Reciprocal innervation:
    interplay between the muscle groups.

4. Normal sensation

Abnormal tone will destroy the balance of the postural reflex mechanism. Imagine what it is like to have no balance reactions. Treatment must involve both sides of the body (make a symmetrical approach), must train body alignment, and must train balance reactions. Abnormal tone includes hypertonus and hypotonus and may involve flexor synergies and extensor synergies with total involvement of the affected side. It is important to treat each patient as an individual and to treat what you find. Therefore careful assessment is necessary; a detailed and carefully recorded test chart ought to be kept and this will serve as a progress report. Assessment of muscle tone, sensory integration and intellect should be made.

A quick early assessment of muscle tone is made in the following way:

The arm. Move the arm into the full inhibiting pattern and note any resistance imposed by spasticity, or for the heavy rag doll effect of loss of tone. Placing is easier the further the limb is away from the dominant abnormal pattern, that is, placing is easier when the limb is moved into the recovery, or inhibiting, pattern. In sitting, arm elevation is more difficult because flexor tone predominates in sitting; thus the arm is best tested and treated in lying and standing and not in sitting.

The leg. Again move into the inhibiting pattern to test tone. This is a straightforward flexion test without allowing the hip to go into outward rotation; the test is also done with the patient lying in supine.

WHY USE MAT WORK?

For two main reasons it is essential to use mat work.

1. Mat work gives the only possible method for following through the sequence of motor development as seen in the human infant until normal controlled movement is regained.

2. Mat work is of particular value to the patient whose stability is poor, that is, the stroke patient, because it provides:
- a wide base
- a low centre of gravity
- a sense of security.

Should the mat be on the floor?

The answer to this question is that it is usually a case of making do with whatever is available. Usually, where the question of cost has to be considered, the mat provided is placed on the floor. A large floor area that can accommodate a number of mats can be very useful, allowing several patients to be treated at the same time. There must be a ready source of pillows and inflatable splints to be used where necessary to stabilise the vital inhibiting patterns that *must be maintained at all times.*

Are there any advantages in having a high mat?

Certainly, particularly in the early days of treatment. A high mat is more readily accessible, making patient handling much easier in the beginning, the area and height being suitable for sitting, for rolling and for training rolling to sitting. It is important to make sure the patient feels safe and not in danger of falling off the high mat onto the floor. The space from the high mat to the floor can seem like a yawning chasm to an early stroke patient.

Simple muscle work using gross patterns of movement involved in trunk rotation make a sound beginning to an advancing exercise programme. The patient is rehabilitated into rotational patterns, the trunk is mobilised into bilateral rotation, the arm into outward rotation with extension of the elbow, wrist and fingers, and the leg into inward rotation with flexion of knee and ankle.

It is important to remember:

1. Stability of the limbs depends on stability of the trunk. It is therefore

unlikely that a patient with an unstable trunk posture will have stability of the limbs. Thus, postural stability of head, neck and trunk are all-important.

2. Postural tone depends on joint compression. With the exception of the stimuli received via the eyes and vestibular apparatus, one of the most powerful stimuli to postural balance and stability is compression, which is normally experienced when the limb or trunk bear weight.

3. The first step in stroke rehabilitation is to stabilise the patient in side-lying. Wherever possible from Day 1 of treatment (or as soon as this is practical) the patient is taught and encouraged to clasp his hands, fingers interlaced, *palms touching*, (again refer to Fig. 6) keeping both hands in the mid-line position and reaching forward at shoulder level, both legs in the crook position. He is then ready to begin learning to roll from side to side and to stabilise in side-lying. But do not wait until he is proficient in rolling to begin stabilising in side-lying.

To stabilise in side-lying the following points should be noted:

1. The patient is carefully positioned in side-lying.

2. Where necessary pillow support is given.

3. The PNF technique of Rhythmical Stabilisation is useful here but at no time must inhibiting positioning be overlooked.

4. Pillow support is withdrawn as improvement takes place.

5. At no time must the therapist exert pressure which leads to unwanted overflow of activity (or associated reactions) increasing the synergic patterns of tonic contraction. For example, where clasped hands, fingers interlaced, elbows extended is used to inhibit the arm, if the palms are not kept firmly in contact, wrist flexion and elbow flexion will develop. With careful positioning and the support of the inflatable arm splint already described it is a simple matter to divert overflow of activity into the low tonal pattern.

6. The patient may be said to be stabilised when he can hold the starting position without outside support.

7. The position of the patient's head must always be taken into account. As far as tonal distribution in the stroke patient is concerned, side-lying is the most neutral position and, therefore, this is the most suitable position for night sleep with the patient lying on his sound side—provided careful positioning with adequate pillow support is given. But, where the patient has not been fully stabilised in the side-lying position and tends to roll backwards, he will spend the night attempting to roll back onto his side and not sleeping, or he will spend the night on his back. Either way he will be spending the night building up excessive and unwanted tone in spasticity patterns. Lying on the back is the position which builds up extensor tone;

attempting to roll onto the side is a flexion pattern and will build up flexor tone in the forearm. This illustrates the need for very careful and vital positioning to be used from the earliest days.

Note on rhythmical stabilisation

Rhythmical Stabilisation is practised by giving steady static contractions of the muscle groups round the trunk or round the joints. In this case, proximal joints first—shoulder and hip. The static contractions are achieved by applying steady manual pressure from therapist to patient, the therapist using such commands as 'Don't let me move you!'. The pressure should be applied *very slowly* and should gradually build up as the muscles respond. A steady static contraction of one group of muscles is immediately followed by a similar contraction of the antagonistic group, no movement being allowed to take place. This is repeated rhythmically.

EARLY EXERCISE

1. As already stated, simple muscle work using gross patterns of movement involved in trunk rotations make a very sound beginning. When the patient has been stabilised in side-lying, from the side-lying position, exercises in *shoulder rolling forwards and backwards* (upper trunk rotation) ought to be started and followed by *hip rolling forwards and backwards* (lower trunk rotation). There is an obvious advantage in stabilising the affected arm with the pressure splint when undertaking these exercises. The splint maintains the elbow, wrist and fingers in extension—the full inhibiting pattern— diverting tonal flow into the extensors and preventing the unwanted build-up of flexor spasticity. With the splinted arm supported across two pillows, after initial supervision, many patients will quickly learn to carry out this exercise for themselves. All possible self-care exercises should be taught.

2. *Rolling from side to side* as already suggested with hands clasped and arms held forward *at, or above, shoulder level,* knees in the crook position. As soon as this exercise is established it is another excellent self-care exercise provided the patient's palms remain in close contact and his elbows are fully extended. This will also ensure that the shoulders are maintained in flexion with protraction (the necessary inhibitory pattern). Again, it is useful to practise the exercise with pressure splint support on the affected arm. The splint is supported with the patient's sound hand. Movement is led by eyes turning, head turning, arms and shoulders turning, and initially the therapist may assist follow through of hips and legs but this will soon follow automatically.

3. *Bridging* from the supine position, the arm splint controlling associated reactions. The exercise consists of lying on the back with both knees flexed and lifting the hips to balance in this position.

4. *Rolling to forearm propping* in the prone position. Rolling is carried out as already described and the patient is taught to carry the roll on over to prop on the forearms. Note that if the hands are clasped, as already taught, and the arms reach forward to shoulder level, the forearms will finish the movement in the correct position—forearms parallel with outward rotation of the shoulders. The elbows should be immediately under the shoulders so that supporting weight is taken from elbows to shoulders. Remembering the need for early stability of head, neck and trunk, the patient should be stabilised in this position at an early date. Suitable pillow support should be used to maintain the corrective leg pattern, i.e., a pillow under the tibia to maintain knee and ankle flexion, or a small inflatable boot may be used on the foot. This will be discussed later in the text. A half-arm splint should be used to control tone in the wrist and fingers while stabilisation in this position is undertaken. Note that the elderly patient with a stiff lower back should roll over onto a pillow which will support the abdominal region and prevent a painful extension of the lumbar spine. During stabilising procedures the therapist will give reasonable resistance to the back of the patient's head as it is lifted back, bringing in neck extension and the tonic neck extension reflex which increases thrust through the inhibited forearms with elbow extension and an increased demand from elbow to shoulder. The prone position with forearm propping is an excellent position in which to work at stabilising the shoulder as well as the upper trunk.

5. *Stabilising head and neck* using the above position 4. All the way through rehabilitation of the stroke patient the position of the head plays an important role. Stimuli received via the eyes, the ears and the neck proprioceptors are all brought into play—as in rolling. It is reasonable then to consider stabilising the head and neck very early in the rehabilitation programme. The therapist may use one of her hands to help support the affected arm in the inhibiting pattern while she uses the other hand for the stabilising techniques. But this is not as effective as inhibiting with pressure splints. Also the use of these splints will leave both of the therapist's hands free to work on progressive patterns.

6. *Rolling to forearm propping* on the affected arm in side-lying and stabilising in this position. Remember that rotating the shoulders over the pelvis inhibits extensor spasticity. Cross facilitation plays a large part in stroke rehabilitation and associated reactions *must* always be diverted into the low tonal patterns. Here the half-arm splint is very useful and this is also a good position in which to assist in stabilising the shoulder. With stroke patients it is necessary to get tone into the shoulder as soon as possible. The best way to get tone into a limb is to put weight through it. Weight must be transmitted through joints which are maintained in their inhibiting patterns.

7. *Stabilising in sitting.* Stabilising in sitting is undertaken as soon as possible in the rehabilitation programme. At this stage if this has not yet

been done then the patient is usually ready for this kind of training. Figure 8 shows the required positioning and, as indicated, lateral stabilising usually demands special attention. The distribution of muscle tone in the patient's affected arm is controlled if the therapist supports and maintains the necessary inhibiting position. This need is better served by the use of the long arm pressure splint which will also set free at least one of the therapist's hands to apply the necessary stabilising pressures to the patient's body. Her other hand may be required to maintain the position of the splinted hand. This is one of the very useful positions for the occupational therapist to adopt, giving occupational tasks using the sound hand in work which will include cross facilitation. There is a great need for physiotherapist and occupational therapist to work together, each backing up what the other is doing.

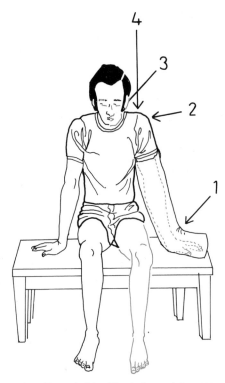

Transferring weight to the affected side. Physiotherapist uses:
1. One hand to maintain patient's hand on the stool.
2. Second hand gives gentle lateral pressure at the shoulder.
3. Gentle pressure to the back of the head to give spinal extension and increase thrust downward in the arms.
4. Increase approximation: pressure downward from the shoulder to the hand.

Fig. 8 Lateral stabilising.

8. *Rolling to forearm propping (as in 6. above) to sitting* and stabilising in sitting is also a valuable exercise sequence, particularly for any elderly patient who is unable to lie in the prone position . *On the floor mat* the patient rolls into side-sitting with his legs in the crook position and propping on his elbow. *On the high mat,* which is more suitable in this situation, the patient rolls to prop on his elbow as he carries his legs over the edge of the mat and comes on up into sitting. Any necessary assistance is given until he can carry out this movement sequence independently. Tonal flow into his affected arm must always be controlled by the inhibitory measures taken by the therapist.

Progress will continue to be made by working forward, stage by stage, to achieve stability in the following positions:

9. *Kneeling with forearm support,* forearms parallel preventing inward rotation of the shoulder (see Fig. 10).

10. *Kneeling with hand support* (see Fig. 9), the crawling position.

11. *High (or stand) kneeling* facing a full-length mirror.

12. *Sitting* as in Figure 8, fully stabilised with no outside support. By this stage a firm placing response with good shoulder protraction has usually been achieved.

13. *Standing.*

Note. **Each advancing starting position must be stabilised**. This is the framework or foundation on which this treatment concept bases its advancing rehabilitation exercise programme. Where the elderly patient is not able to follow this developmental pattern because of a rigid lumbar spine, osteoarthritis of the knees etc., the developmental pattern of rolling to sitting to standing is used.

Each advancing position must be stabilised

The skilled therapist will fully understand and practise the wide variety of therapeutic movements which may be used with each progression. But, during the progressions and with all exercise routines, the therapist must understand, feel with her hands, and see in her mind's eye the total tonal patterns that will result with every movement and must take appropriate measures to inhibit and divert tone as necessary.

For example, consider the bridging position (3. above), lying on the back in the crook position, both knees are bent, feet firmly on the mat, arms out to the sides with shoulders in outward rotation and elbows straight, the necessary inhibiting pattern in the affected arm will be maintained by use of the long arm splint. The total body is now in the total inhibiting pattern. This position will usually not be maintained until the affected hip and leg have been stabilised in the crook position. To begin with, the affected leg will usually flop into outward rotation of the hip and extension of the leg—

this spasticity pattern being set by the strong thrust of *Gluteus maximus*. With the assistance of the therapist, work on the lower trunk and the hip will be used to stabilise the hip in the crook position. The therapist assists in maintaining the starting position by holding both of the patient's knees closely together while lower trunk rotations are undertaken, the movement taking the flexed knees as far as possible in an arc from side to side. This has three distinctly therapeutic effects:

1. It maintains mobility in the lower trunk.
2. It reduces any unwanted antigravity tone in the affected leg.
3. It produces strong overflow of tone into the affected arm which will be diverted into the low tonal pattern because of the total inhibiting pattern imposed by the long arm splint.

Next, using the basic crook lying position, the therapist will further stabilise the affected leg by assisting movement into inward rotation of the hip until this becomes a voluntary exercise and then an exercise which can be done against resistance. Rhythmical stabilisation is also useful here. Still using the long arm splint, as soon as the starting position is thoroughly stabilised the patient is ready to do the bridging exercise unassisted. This is a vital progression because the patient will spend many hours sitting in a chair which includes hip flexion—this is the inhibiting hip pattern *but hip extension must not be lost*. The patient who remains unable to bridge will never again regain a good walking gait.

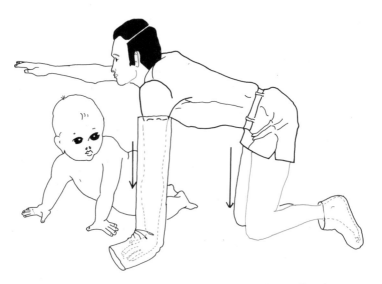

Fig. 9   The crawling pattern. Weightbearing through the affected arm.

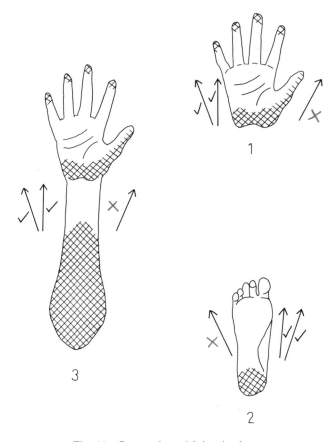

Fig. 10   Correct the weightbearing bases.

In all the progressions in treatment sustained pressure splints may be used to maintain inhibiting limb positions and to supply stability.

This has led to the development of a range of suitable splints—see Chapter 5.

Weightbearing on a limb increases muscle tone. Therefore it should be noted that the position of the weightbearing base of the limb is important because this position will affect the distribution of the tone in the limb above. A study of Figure 10, where arrows are used to indicate the necessary weightbearing bases for hemiplegic limbs, is helpful.

Position 1

Weightbearing through the hand illustrates the need to place the hand pointing straight forward or outwardly to ensure that the shoulder joint above is maintained in outward rotation. This will help to increase the required shoulder tone and will not increase the unwanted antigravity tone.

Position 2

Weightbearing on the foot, weight must be transmitted through the heel with the foot pointing straight forward or into inward rotation and *not* through the front of an outwardly rotated foot. This is to ensure that *Gluteus maximus* is not contributing to a strong antigravity thrust.

Position 3

Weightbearing through the forearm and hand, the forearm points straight forward or into outward rotation, again to make sure the shoulder joint is not allowed to weightbear in the antigravity pattern of inward rotation.

By observing these simple rules an important factor in the recovery of normal movement has been taken into account in the designing of the necessary pressure splints to support the treatment programme and is an integral part of the basic concept.

It should be noted that in Figure 10 you are looking at the weightbearing base from below.

4. Assessment

MUSCLE TONE AND THE STROKE PATIENT: THE IMPORTANCE OF ASSESSMENT

Because there is always an alteration from normal to abnormal muscle tone in the stroke patient, it is important to assess this factor with great care. Rehabilitation consists of finding the abnormal and attempting to shift it back to normal. This assessment cannot be undertaken without understanding the following points—far less can an effective treatment be offered.

1. Normal tone

Defined as the normal resistance offered to a passive movement in the absence of any other muscle or joint disease.

2. Resting tone

The tone required to maintain the position of a limb or part of the body against gravity.

3. Dynamic tone

The tone required to maintain the position of a limb during normal activity.

4. Placing

A term that ought to be understood. The normal human being has the ability to 'place' a limb. This means he can maintain a limb in space in any position. The ability to do this may be lost where there is a change in tone, for example, the stroke patient's limb will usually drift into the dominant reflex pattern—the pattern of spasticity.

Changes in normal tone come under three headings

1. *Hypertonicity* or spastic paralysis, muscle spasm, spasticity. The limb will drift at all times into the total pattern of spasticity and will be resistant to movement into the recovery, or normal movement pattern when handled by another person.

2. *Hypotonicity* or flaccid paralysis, muscle weakness. The patient will have lost his placing response, he will be unable to support the limb against gravity and it will feel heavy and abnormally relaxed if handled by another person.

3. *Tremor,* usually referred to as intention tremor. Here the patient will be unable to hold a position in space and in cerebellar lesions he will be quite unable to hold the total antigravity position. He will drift when he attempts to hold and overshoot when he moves.

When treating stroke patients it is often found that more than one of these changes in normal muscle tone may be present in any one patient and symptoms co-exist. The skill of the physiotherapist lies in her ability to make a sound assessment and treat according to her findings. Where she works hand in hand with an occupational therapist she should pass on her findings (as should the occupational therapist where she does assessment of cognitive or perceptual difficulty).

Techniques used to decrease muscle tone may include:

1. *Positioning* in inhibiting patterns. It is found in practice in the clinical field that this is an essential part of all stroke care.

2. *Pressure splints,* orally inflated enclosing a limb in the total inhibitory (or recovery) pattern to inhibit dominant reflexes.

3. *Passive movements.*

4. *Active assisted movements* where the physiotherapist maintains the initiative. Movements keep within the recovery pattern and pay particular attention to shoulder and hip positioning.

5. *Active assisted movements* where the patient may begin to take the initiative provided the recovery pattern is fully maintained so that the dominant reflexes are fully inhibited. Here the pressure splint assists an early approach to active work.

6. *Weightbearing over a correctly positioned base* with the pressure splint supplying stability.

7. *The skilful use of reflex activity.*

Techniques used to increase muscle tone may include:

1. *Use of an orally inflatable pressure splint* to support the limb in the recovery (the full inhibitory) pattern while exercising the proximal joint, e.g. the shoulder joint.

2. *Sustained, superficial and deep pressure.* Again, with use of the pressure splint to give sustained pressure while movement within the tissues is stimulated (e.g. by rolling from side to side).

3. *Approximation of joint surfaces,* with supporting assistance of the pressure splint to give stability and to maintain the inhibiting pattern while exercises in limb loading, or weightbearing, are used to facilitate underlying postural mechanisms.

4. *Intermittent pressure to soft tissues* given with the assistance of a mechanical pump to a limb enclosed in a pressure splint.

5. *Active assisted movements* leading to holding in space and often made possible at an early date because of the sustained posture offered by the sustained pressure splint.

6. *Tapping (or pounding)* of the heel of the patient's foot, or the heel of his hand, with the limb held in the inhibiting pattern.

7. *Weightbearing* over a correctly positioned base.

8. *The skilful use of reflex activity.*

SUMMARY OF REFLEX ACTIVITY

1. *Tonic reflexes* are reflexes which produce involuntary changes in muscle tone in response to stimulation of sensory nerve endings—exteroceptors and proprioceptors. Of these we are most concerned with stimulation of the proprioceptors in response to changes of the body's position in space giving pressure on soft tissues, for example in rolling, and in weight transference. There are three distinct types of response:

(a) *The positive supporting response.* This gives an increase in extensor tone in a limb bearing weight.

(b) *The negative supporting response.* This gives a decrease in extensor tone when weight is taken off a limb.

(c) *The withdrawal response.* This response does not need consideration in stroke rehabilitation except perhaps for the relatively uncommon flexor withdrawal of the hemiplegic leg. (See Chapter 5, application of the leg gaiter, Method B.) It is a very rapid response which takes place as a result of painful stimuli to give an increase in flexor tone.

These are all involuntary reflex happenings but should be understood if re-education of the postural reflex mechanism is to be undertaken.

2. *Righting reflexes.* A combination of righting reflexes makes up a righting response, or the appropriate response which leads to equilibrium. They may be recognised under three distinct headings:

(a) *The head righting response.* This follows movement of the head in space with correction of eye level in response to disturbance of the labyrinth.

(b) *Head, neck and trunk response.* The head rights, movement of the cervical spine stretches the neck muscles and triggers off the reflex mechanism to bring the body into alignment of head, neck and trunk.

(c) *Rotation response.* This gives the ability to rotate within the body axis.

A study of these reflexes makes very sound sense of following neurodevelopmental patterns in stroke rehabilitation. So far so good, but it is also necessary to study equilibrium responses. Equilibrium responses follow in the development patterns and are much more complex. It should be understood that they develop from righting responses.

3. *Equilibrium responses,* as just stated, follow in the development pattern. Tonic reflexes, which give changes in muscle tone with weight transference, combine with righting responses to give automatic shifts in tone all over the body which relate to position changes, making possible the patterns of movement necessary for daily living. Equilibrium responses may also be placed under three headings:

(a) *Automatic shifts of tone*
   (i) In response to changing centre of gravity.
   (ii) When 'placing' a limb, to maintain 'place'.
   (iii) When resting (= resting tone).

(b) *Movements of compensation to allow the body to support its weight over a fixed base.*
   (i) The propping response.
   (ii) Magnet reactions—an equal and balancing weight—counterpoise.

(c) *Movements of compensation to allow the body to find a necessary new supporting base.*
   (i)   The stepping response.
   (ii) The hopping response.
   (iii) The protective response, for example, extension of the arms.

So, equilibrium responses include shifts in muscle tone with compensating movements to allow the body to stand up to any alterating situation that may be caused by changes in position or environment. When fully developed, equilibrium responses make it possible for us to support our weight over a fixed base while reaching out in any direction, to maintain balance against an external opposing force, or to regain lost balance by stepping, hopping or reaching out.

As has already been stated, tonic responses are stereotyped primitive responses which are modified at higher levels when the postural reflex mechanism is fully established. But it is important to note that righting and equilibrium responses probably include a cortical element and are variable. They may be modified or overruled at cortical level.

Where the antigravity responses that are necessary *to control and maintain equilibrium* are missing, there can be no normal control of posture and no normal patterns of movement.

Conclusion

To undertake stroke rehabilitation and so to set out to restore the postural reflex mechanism the four levels of reflex activity must be understood. To follow the development of this reflex mechanism is to follow through these four stages. I have covered this subject more fully elsewhere.* To understand the basic need of the stroke patient is to understand the urgent need to restore normal muscle tone. This cannot be done without understanding the levels of reflex activity. Assessment of the patient's state of muscle tone must be given first priority.

ACCURATE ASSESSMENT AND REHABILITATION

To establish the importance of accurate assessment in the rehabilitation programme, look first at the missing function facing the patient:

1. Loss of normal muscle tone.
2. Developing spasticity.
3. Sensory disturbance.
4. Loss of normal movement.

Because of this missing function the patient is faced with:

1. Lack of rotation.
2. No adaptation to gravity.
3. No gradation of movement.
4. No protective extension.
5. **Balance** is missing.

Looking again at the missing function, the two factors contributing to the loss of normal movement are lack of **Inhibition** and lack of **Normal Sensation,** so why not follow infant developmental patterns? From the primitive reflex movement present at birth, using movement patterns that are familiar to all of us, the infant works up through the levels of reflex activity until cortical control is established. These reflex levels ought to be understood so that the various responses may be correctly applied during rehabilitation of the stroke patient in any attempt to restore normal muscle tone. These responses are:

---

* *Restoration of Motor Function in the Stroke Patient,* Churchill Livingstone, 1987, Third Edition.

1. **Spinal**. Spinal reflex level/involuntary changes in muscle tone.
2. **Tonic**. Mid-brain responses/tonic neck reflexes/labyrinthine reflexes.
3. **Basal**. Righting reflexes/equilibrium responses.
4. **Cortical**. Voluntary responses.*

A study of the above facts would seem to confirm the need to follow movement patterns used by the infant. The infant incorporates head movements and rolling patterns at an early stage of development. Is this not exactly what is needed in stroke rehabilitation? *Rolling patterns are flexion patterns*. The stroke patient has an urgent need to be taught a way of inhibiting the developing spasticity patterns which are extension antigravity patterns. The use of rolling patterns will usually answer the patient's needs, flexion for the total body—*except for the elbow, wrist and fingers*. It is this fact alone which is largely responsible for failure to rehabilitate a useful functioning arm in the hemiplegic patient. A way has to be found of successfully inhibiting flexor tone in the forearm. Find a way to fully maintain the necessary inhibitory pattern of extension in the elbow, wrist and fingers, *diverting tonal flow into extension*, and then start with rolling patterns.

There are a few who do not agree with the approach to rehabilitation which is presented here. But the success or failure of any rehabilitation approach must surely be based on the results achieved in the clinical field. I would suggest that a clinical trial over a number of years where a rehabilitation concept is faithfully put into practice with careful observation and recording of the results achieved can be the only true judge of the validity of any theory. These results must make the final analysis. I undertook just such a study in an acute hospital over a period of eight years. The rehabilitation principles set out in this book were faithfully followed in every detail (including the need for vigilant positioning, early treatment and constant repetition of movements within inhibiting patterns) and the recorded results were very satisfactory. This, in my mind, is sufficient to establish the validity of any rehabilitation concept. We are talking about restoring motor control and, in many cases, to the restoration of a fully working hand with the return of skilled precision movements. I should also state that this was a team effort which included rehabilitation nurses trained in the necessary round-the-clock inhibitory positioning.

It is important to remember that the patient's needs will be established by accurate assessment. Also, the factors responsible for muscle tone are the cerebral cortex or other higher cerebral region, the vestibular nucleus, the spinal cord, the muscle spindle and the anterior horn cell of the spinal cord. The aim of treatment is to give back to the brain-damaged patient inhib-

---

* For a more detailed account refer to *Restoration of Motor Function in the Stroke Patient*, Margaret Johnstone, Churchill Livingstone, 1987, Third Edition.

itory control over abnormal patterns of movement. The purpose of treatment is to restore postural control.

Given these facts, the first priority of the physiotherapist in the clinical field is to understand the normal, to understand the disruption of the normal in her stroke patients and then to go straight to the heart of the main rehabilitation problem by making an accurate assessment of the patient's state of muscle tone. Almost without exception in rehabilitation this is step number one.

I am convinced that reliable assessment of the state of muscle tone is not a skill that can be taught in the classroom; it is an ability that can only be taught and developed in the clinical field with a hands-on approach until the student is able to use techniques to divert, shift and therapeutically use tonal patterns to meet the needs of the individual patient. The physiotherapist *feels* the patient's tonal distribution, examines the tonal patterns when she stimulates extra tonal input by bringing in head movements, or she promotes overflow of tone which is stimulated by movements of the sound half of the body. (Such a simple action as yawning will frequently be seen to step up unwanted flexor tone in the forearm.)

A provisional and quick assessment of the patient's tonal state may be made by moving a disabled limb into the total inhibiting pattern. Where spasticity (or hypertonicity) is present, the further the limb is passively moved into this inhibitory pattern the more resistant it becomes. The limb will drift at all times into the total pattern of spasticity and will be resistant to movement into the inhibiting pattern *when handled by another person.* On the other hand, where the limb gives no resistance but is heavy to handle (the floppy doll limb) flaccidity (or hypotonicity) is present. The patient will have lost his placing response, he will be unable to support the limb against gravity and it will feel heavy and abnormally relaxed if handled by another person. In stroke rehabilitation it is important to remember that even the flaccid limb will eventually show signs of developing spasticity which is usually first noted in the fingers. Therefore it is important to use careful positioning in inhibitory patterns from the early days and to practise the special pressure techniques necessary to put tone into the limb.

A more detailed and accurate assessment will be made in the following way. With the patient lying in the supine position, the lower half of his body is carefully placed and supported with pillows in a relaxed inhibitory pattern while the arm is tested. Grading may be made by numbers of 1 to 5, 5 representing normal and associated reactions will be nil. Six tests to grade the state of muscle tone may be given:

1. Can the patient hold his arm in elevation (vertical), it having been placed there?

2. Can he lower the extended arm through abduction from elevation to horizontal?

3. Can he return the arm to position 1?

4. With his arm in elevation, can he bend his elbow to touch the top of his head in supination?

5. Can he return the arm to position 4 staying in supination?

6. Can he extend the arm in elevation with outward rotation while he carries out grasp and release exercise with his hand?

It will be noted from these tests that from 1 to 5 gets progressively more difficult. Number 6 represents the normal. To give an example, when undertaking test number 1 the physiotherapist will place the patient's arm in elevation (without considering joint rotation) simply to see if he is able to maintain this placed position. In many cases in the early days of treatment the patient cannot maintain even this fairly simple position, regardless of the shoulder pattern. At once the physiotherapist understands the need to apply the long arm splint in the fully inhibiting pattern for the elbow, wrist and fingers, giving the arm the necessary stability while *work on the trunk is undertaken*.

The grading scale should be charted with care. Further explanation of the grading numbers will help to establish the accuracy of advancing tests. For example, to give a test a grade of 0 is self-explanatory. Grade 1 will indicate some control of proximal joints. If, between tests, there has been some slight improvement but the patient's muscle tone is not considered to have reached grade 2, the physiotherapist may indicate the improvement on the chart by writing 1+. If the former ability has decreased, 1− will be given. Wherever possible the same therapist should carry out initial and all subsequent tests.

Notes on this scale of grading:

1. Some control of proximal joints.
2. As in 1, but with independent movement possible in middle joints.
3. As in 2, but with independent movement possible in distal joints.
4. Good control, individual movement of distal joints but with some abnormal tonal pattern on reinforcement.
5. Normal.

SENSORY LOSS AND THE STROKE PATIENT: THE IMPORTANCE OF ASSESSMENT

Sensory loss may be a major barrier to rehabilitation and an early estimate of any disability in this area should be made. Postural sense, vision, sensation and abstract thought should be assessed as soon as possible. There are four initial and very quick tests which may be used to indicate any sensory deficit in these areas. I have frequently found these tests most useful and I am grateful to Professor Bernard Isaacs who gave them to me with his free permission to use them.

1. Postural sense

Ask the patient to grasp the thumb of his affected hand with his sound hand. Repeat the task with the eyes covered but the position of the affected arm is altered after the eyes are covered. The patient with defective proprioception will fail to find his thumb.

2. Vision

Hemianopia and visual agnosia must not be confused (agnosia—loss of the power to perceive). Neglect of one half of space is very quickly demonstrated when two brightly coloured pens of contrasting colours are held in front of the patient about 12 inches apart and he fails to identify one of them.

Note. The patient with hemianopia will only see one pen but he will see both pens if they are interchanged in front of his eyes because he is able to follow the pen that moves into the blind half of his visual field. In cases of severe neglect of half of space, only one pen is seen even when they are moved so that they are in front of the patient and less than one inch apart. Even when they are interchanged in front of the patient's eyes he will not be able to follow the pen that moves into the blind half of his visual field.

3. Sensation

Cutaneous sensibility, or tactile sensation, ought to be tested. Identify light touch on any part of the body without the help of the eyes. Two-point discrimination is also used, the result of the test depending on the patient's ability to distinguish two points from one on the finger pulps without using the eyes.

4. Abstract thought

Use a quick test*, e.g. *Picture identification*. The test suggested here will also uncover visual agnosia and neglect of the left half of space and takes no

---

* With a little practice none of these tests take more than a minute. They give a very quick initial assessment of brain damage usually associated with the non-dominant lobe and indicate the need to make a sound sensorimotor approach to rehabilitation.

For a full account of assessment possibilities consult my book *Restoration of Motor Function in the Stroke Patient*, Churchill Livingstone, 1987, Third Edition.

more than a minute in time. A picture of a man and a woman is all that is needed, preferably a bride and groom, and the picture should be mounted for easy handling. The patient is shown the picture and asked a series of questions:

'What do you see?'

If he cannot identify the picture he is asked:

'Is there a man in the picture?'

'Point to the man!'

'Is there anyone else?'

'Is there a woman?'

'Point to the woman.'

'What is the woman wearing?' . . . and so on.

Interpretation of the test:

(a) Patients with visual agnosia fail completely.

(b) Patients with neglect of the left half of space fail to identify the figure in the left half of the picture.

(c) Patients with loss of abstract thought fail to give a general interpretation of the picture, e.g. they call the bride a 'woman' or misidentify the picture because they misinterpret a fundamental detail, e.g. the bride may be described as a nurse.

Drawing tests

Where sensorimotor disturbance is present it is an established fact that, where the non-dominant hemisphere is involved, the difficulties facing rehabilitation may be severe. No two stroke patients present exactly the same problems. It is always necessary to carry out very careful and therefore accurate assessment of the damage resulting from the individual stroke. It is also important to remember that performance will vary from day to day and, where severe damage is present, a reliable assessment for future prognosis cannot be made in the early days. Indeed, it will be a full month after onset before a prognosis assessment (with no sensory involvement) may be in any way reliable. Over many years, in my clinical studies, I have come to believe that all stroke patients have some degree of sensory loss—but I may have reached this conclusion because most of my time over a period of 25 years has been taken up with the severely brain-damaged patient. Where sensory involvement is included the time necessary to reach a reliable prognosis assessment will usually be at least 2 months. If parietal lobe syndrome is included, the prognosis assessment time will be 3 to 4 months. These figures depend on intensive treatment with correct handling.

Drawing tests are frequently used to assist in making an accurate assessment but these tests must be interpreted correctly. The following notes will help:

Interpretation of drawings which should be done on a separate sheet of paper for each drawing using a felt-tipped pen and a firm clip-board.

1. Make allowances for left-handed drawings by the right-handed patient.
2. Always note the position of the drawing on the page, remembering that patients with neglect of the left half of space place their drawings on the right half of the page.
3. Note the size of the drawing, remembering that demented patients tend to make a very small drawing.
4. An elaborate detailed drawing tends to point to a high intellectual level prior to the stroke.
5. Note the placing of the parts of the body which will be disrupted, grossly misshapen, or missing in cases of agnosia.
6. Leaving out the left half of a drawing, for example a house, indicates visual agnosia, or severe neglect of the left half of space.
7. Incoherent drawing usually indicates receptive dysphasia or dyspraxia; repetitive scribbling should be noted as perseveration.
8. The drawing with a lateral lean, or the progressive lateral lean of repeated arrows drawn across a page, may indicate postural difficulties. A vertical arrow pointing upwards and not too small is drawn on the left side of the sheet of paper and the patient is asked to copy the arrow right across the page.
9. The clock with numbers wandering outside the face indicates general brain damage—as distinct from the clock with numbers omitted in cases of spatial neglect.

Draw a man, draw a house, and **draw a clock** are the subjects most frequently used in these tests. **Copy drawings** of these same subjects are very useful tests, particularly where **agnosia, apraxia** or **spatial neglect** on either side is suspected. Drawings to be copied ought to be done by the therapist in front of the patient. The drawing should then be moved upward so that it is immediately *above* the sheet of paper and not alongside it. Always stress that the ability to draw well does not matter. Always remember that each new drawing must be done on a fresh piece of paper and one drawing is completed before the next is attempted. Always sit quietly and watch the patient's performance. Decide whose responsibility it is to conduct these tests; in a well integrated team it is usually considered to be the occupational therapist's task but all therapists ought to be competent enough to undertake all tests. Avoid the mistake which is made when one therapist conducts the drawing tests and then the patient moves on to the next department where the tests are immediately repeated because the so-called stroke team is not fully integrated! Information about patient assessment, treatment, progress etc. must pass freely between team members and team members should be prepared to share their expertise, to cross another's borders and truly integrate to produce a satisfactory treatment programme which is in the best interest of the individual patient.

Figures 11 and 12 give examples of assessment tests which are not difficult to interpret and clearly show neglect of the left half of space. With intensive treatment using pressure techniques including intermittent pressure the patient made a satisfactory recovery.

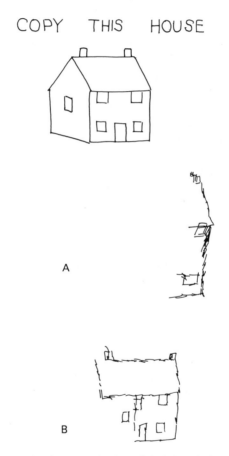

Fig. 11 Drawing test showing severe neglect of the left half of space: A = copy of house 4 weeks after onset of stroke; B = copy of house 8 weeks after onset of stroke. From A to B all pressure techniques were used.

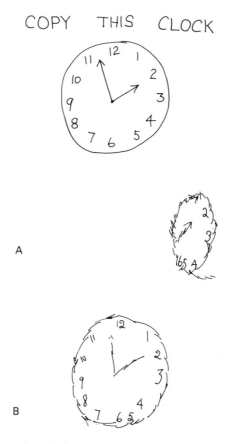

Fig. 12   Drawing test done by the same patient as in Figure 11 and at the same time.

Assessment must include:

1. The state of muscle tone.
2. Motor loss.
3. Sensory loss.
4. Parietal lobe involvement.
5. Hearing.
6. Vision.
7. Communication difficulty. *Note.* Here the assessment and advice of the speech therapist is essential in many cases (see below).

Parietal lobe involvement

Assessment becomes relatively less difficult if this is understood. It is helpful to divide the possible defects of hemispheres under two headings:

Dominant hemisphere	*Non-dominant hemisphere*
1. Bilateral apraxia	1. Constructional apraxia
2. Tactile astereognosis	2. Tactile astereognosis
3. Postural difficulties	3. Postural difficulties
4. Right/left disorientation	4. Disorder of spatial judgment
5. Finger agnosia	5. Visual agnosia
6. Dysgraphia	6. Anosognosia—neglect or denial of ownership of limbs
7. Dyscalculia	7. Disturbance of body image

Visual defects

1. Loss of field (hemianopia)
2. Agnosia (difficulty in recognition)
3. Inattention (inability to channel visual input)
4. Visuo-spatial disturbance
5. Visual scanning (series of letters given, failure to pick out all O's)
6. Visual spanning (more complex instruction, e.g. cancel out D when it occurs after E)
7. *Neglect of half of space* must be distinguished from visual loss of field = hemianopia.

A breakdown in communication (speech, reading and writing)

As already stated, where there are communication difficulties the speech therapist's assessment may be of vital importance. There may be hidden difficulties which are not apparent to other members of the stroke team which can cause the patient great distress if they are not uncovered or *understood* (this includes nurses and family members). These can only be dealt with by the skilled expert—the speech therapist.

In all three of the 1987 editions of my books* I have attempted to deal with some of the communication problems but probably the best contribution comes from the expert herself—an experienced senior speech therapist with her contribution to the *Home Care* book. As this book is aimed at bringing understanding to the lay person, the speech therapy section is written at this level but is very useful for all other team members. Without the basic understanding presented here, therapists and nurses will not understand the speech therapist's findings nor will they be able to carry out her instructions with a reasonable hope of doing as she asks.

---

* *Home Care for the Stroke Patient*, 1987, Second Edition.
  The Stroke Patient—A Team Approach, 1987, Third Edition.
  Restoration of Motor Function in the Stroke Patient, 1987, Third Edition. All published by Churchill Livingstone.

Where there are not enough speech therapists to have one in each rehabilitation unit, at least it is hopefully possible to be able to call on an expert to assess the patient and then to give advice to the rest of the team on how to approach the patient—or, sometimes more importantly, how *not* to approach the patient, e.g. it is wrong to expect the dysphasic patient to have the ability to use a communication chart.

I can only repeat the urgent need to include a skilled speech therapist in any rehabilitation situation offered to the patient with a breakdown in communication or any suspected problems that come within the speech therapist's area. This need may be met by having just one such therapist who is not a resident member of a complete working unit but who may be *called in to visit and make the necessary assessments in the hospital or* **home situation**. If expert follow-up treatments are judged to be necessary the shortage of skilled speech therapists can still cause problems.

An assessment chart should be used in all rehabilitation situations. Figures 13, 14 and 15 illustrate the chart that I have found to be the most useful in recent years.

Figure 16 gives an example of the first page of the chart which was used over a period of approximately 3 months. The patient concerned has been given a fictitious name. During his 3 months in the hospital stroke unit a family member came twice weekly to assist at treatment sessions and was successfully instructed in continuing home care. With his discharge home a visiting therapist supervised his home care by visiting once a week and later reported a very satisfactory rehabilitation outcome. Visiting therapist and family continued to use pressure splints and pressure techniques until hand recovery was complete.

Look again at Figure 16 and note that it is almost entirely devoted to **gross motor performance**. One glance at this and it will be seen not only as an **assessment of motor performance** but also as a detailed **progress report**. The red circles have been added to pinpoint the remaining disability at the time he went home and to emphasise the areas which still need to have special attention during exercise sessions. This copy of the assessment chart which I used in my stroke unit is a typical example. All patients admitted to the unit had failed to rehabilitate elsewhere and had been classed as not expected to make any significant recovery!

Note. Whatever the method chosen to record assessment findings and a treatment programme, careful records should be kept and treatment progress noted. Set realistic goals and adjust the programme to meet any changing situation. Much will depend on the therapist's cheerful approach and the rapport established between the patient and his helpers (therapists, doctors, nurses and family members).

NAME .... AGE ....

DIAGNOSIS .... OCCUPATION ....

DATE OF ONSET .... WARD...

DATE OF ADMISSION .... DATE OF DISCHARGE ....

MUSCLE TONE: Are the limbs resistant to the following movements or are they
heavy and abnormally relaxed?

DATE

ARM movement into recovery pattern
      plus elevation.

LEG movement into recovery pattern plus
      full flexion.

(State: Resistant or Heavy = Spastic or Flaccid = S1, 2, 3 or Fl, 2, 3.)

GROSS MOTOR PERFORMANCE: IN BED DATE

1. Roll from supine to right
2. Roll from supine to left
3. Bridging
4. Roll to elbow propping
5. Roll to sitting over edge of bed
6. Sitting without use of hands
7. Transfer from bed to chair

GROSS MOTOR PERFORMANCE: IN PHYSIO.

1. Rolling to prone lying
2. Prone lying with forearm support
3. Kneeling with forearm support
4. Full kneeling to stand kneeling
5. Crawling

GROSS MOTOR PERFORMANCE: BALANCE

1. In sitting
2. In kneeling
3. In standing

GROSS MOTOR PERFORMANCE: WEIGHT
TRANSFERS

1. Over affected hip in sitting
2. Over affected hand in sitting
3. Cross R leg over L in sitting
4. Cross L leg over R in sitting
5. Sitting to standing with hands clasped
6. Over affected hip in standing
7. Controlled walking.

Scale of grading:- 3—unaided, 2—with minimal help, 1—with help, 0—impossible.

Fig. 13

Record returning normal muscle tone

SUPINE upper limb. Grade 1–5 5 = Normal, associated reactions nil.

1. Patient holding extended arm in elevation, arm
   vertical, it having been placed there.

2. Lower the extended arm through abduction from
   elevation to horizontal.

3. Return.

4. With extended arm in elevation, bend elbow to
   touch top of head in supination.

5. Return in supination.

6. Hold extended arm in elevation, in lateral rotation,
   grasp and release.

SUPINE lower limb.

1. Affected leg flexed and foot resting, keep knee in
   mid-line. (Yes or No)

2. From extension, flex hip in mid-line to more than
   90° with dorsiflexed foot.

3. Return to extension maintaining dorsiflexed foot.
                                              DATE

Scale of grading:

1 — some control of proximal joints

2 — as in 1, but with independent movement
    possible in middle joints

3 — as in 2, but with independent movement
    possible in distal joints

4 — good control, individual movement of
    distal joints but with some abnormal
    tonal pattern on reinforcement

5 — normal

Fig. 14

Cortical integration and sensory interpretation—tactile and postural sensitivity: tested with eyes covered.

DATE								
Pin-prick								
Joint position								
Light touch								
Two point								
Size and texture								

Fill in: PASSES, FAILED or UNCERTAIN

Test for hemianopia:

Draw a Man:

Where 'Draw a Man' fails, give the test *Copy a Man*

DATE		
Copy a Man:		
Copy a Clock:		
Copy a House:		

Above tests to uncover NEGLECT, AGNOSIA and APRAXIA

DATE		
Mental Capacity: How does the patient answer simple questions?		

Any other medical history to be considered during rehabilitation?

Social background?

Any other relevant comments?

Fig. 15

NAME JACKSON, GEORGE   AGE Date of Birth 29/12/1910

DIAGNOSIS C.V.A. (L—R DISABILITY IS   OCCUPATION Retired
          LEFT HANDED)

DATE OF ONSET JULY 1984   WARD 2

DATE OF ADMISSION SEPTEMBER 1984   DATE OF DISCHARGE Home 2nd
                                        JANUARY 1985

MUSCLE TONE: Are the limbs resistant to the following movements or are they
            heavy and abnormally relaxed? Heavy

2 months post stroke
↓   4 months post stroke
             ↓   ↓ 5 months post stroke

	Test 1	Test 2	Test 3		
ARM movement into recovery pattern plus elevation.	F2	F1	Balanced		
LEG movement into recovery pattern plus full flexion.	F1	F1	Balanced		

(State: Resistant or Heavy = Spastic or Flaccid = S1, 2, 3 or Fl, 2, 3.)

GROSS MOTOR PERFORMANCE: IN BED

	Test 1	Test 2	Test 3	Home	Care
1. Roll from supine to right	2	3	3		
2. Roll from supine to left	1	3	3		
3. Bridging	1	3	3		
4. Roll to elbow propping	0	2	3		
5. Roll to sitting over edge of bed	0	1+	(2+)		
6. Sitting without use of hands	2	3	3		
7. Transfer from bed to chair	1	3	3		

GROSS MOTOR PERFORMANCE: IN PHYSIO.

	Test 1	Test 2	Test 3		
1. Rolling to prone lying	0	2	3		
2. Prone lying with forearm support	0	2+	3		
3. Kneeling with forearm support	0	3	3		
4. Full kneeling to stand kneeling	0	2	3		
5. Crawling	0	1+	(2)		

Fig. 16

GROSS MOTOR PERFORMANCE: BALANCE

1. In sitting	2	3	3	
2. In kneeling	0	2	3	
3. In standing	0	1+	(2)	

GROSS MOTOR PERFORMANCE: WEIGHT TRANSFERS

1. Over affected hip in sitting	0	3	3	
2. Over affected hand in sitting	0	2	(2+)	
3. Cross R leg over L in sitting	0	2	3	
4. Cross L leg over R in sitting	0	3	3	
5. Sitting to standing with hands clasped	0	2+	3	
6. Over affected hip in standing	0	1	(2)	
7. Controlled walking.	0	1	(1+)	

Scale of grading:- 3—unaided, 2—with minimal help, 1—with help, 0—impossible.

Fig. 16 (*contd*)

5. An update on pressure splints

Returning to the neurological background on which the stroke rehabilitation programme is built, and considering the brain damage sustained in the majority of stroke victims, two factors necessary for successful rehabilitation have become of first importance.

1. The need to inhibit the stretch reflex where the inhibitory input from the brain is lacking.
2. The need to step up sensory input where there is sensory loss.

Failure to adequately supply these two major needs combined with the frequent lack of *early treatment* led to failed rehabilitation and the crippling disabilities of residual problems with little hope of a return to an acceptable quality of life. Despair was the frequent outcome for the stroke victim. On the other hand, rehabilitation can often be surprisingly straightforward if *treatment begins early* after the onset of the stroke and if the necessary inhibitory control and sensory input are dynamic.

Pressure techniques resulted from a long study of 25 years in which I worked in the clinical field seeking answers to these two main barriers to rehabilitation.

The need to control excessive tone and to shift tonal flow into inhibiting patterns needed considerably more than the laying on of a therapist's hands for a short (usually all too short) session each day. Corrective positioning gave some sort of answer. The patient was taught the necessary inhibitory patterns where possible, if he was lucky, and the correct furniture was used so that these inhibiting positions might be maintained during resting periods. But this had proved far from adequate. A strong outside influence on tonal patterns plus considerably longer rehabilitation sessions seemed to be necessary. For example, where rehabilitation was concerned, one of the early and essential needs for the hemiplegic arm was to get tone into the subluxed or weak shoulder. The best way to push in the necessary tone would be achieved by putting weight through the joint *but* this had to be done putting weight through the shoulder using the inhibiting antigravity pattern. The long arm inflatable pressure splint which ambulance men were using seemed to answer this need. The splint was applied to give the limb stability and to maintain the inhibitory pattern of extension in the elbow, wrist and fingers. Then, using the hand as the weightbearing base and correctly positioned in outward rotation, the required tone would be pushed in to work towards stabilising the shoulder. In the clinical field it soon became apparent that the use of this splint was also going a long way towards answering the second priority, the need to step up sensory input.

Early weightbearing through the arm gave a very positive sensory boost through the joint proprioceptors. Next, in the acute hospital where strokes were admitted on Day 1 of onset and with a nursing team trained in corrective positioning and the urgent need to carry out this corrective positioning 24 hours a day, use of this pressure splint, in many cases, was giving unexpectedly excellent results in arm rehabilitation. The use of the arm splint was incorporated into treatment sessions wherever missing inhibition from the brain had disrupted reciprocal inhibition. Carefully handled it seemed possible to keep arm recovery just ahead of leg recovery and to finally achieve a working hand capable of precision and skilled function. Average time as an inpatient was 1 month and follow-up as an outpatient for 2 months.

Note. Unfortunately it is difficult to achieve such an ideal set up in the present day, frequently understaffed hospitals. Also it appears in many nursing schools there is little or no neurological education and nurses do not understand the major role they could play in motor recovery for the hemiplegic patient. 'We haven't got time!', a nurse may say. But, if she understood her role in the rehabilitation team, such as therapeutic resting positions (see Fig. 17), she would find that it is much easier and quicker to follow out nursing procedures if she observes the simple handling principles that are required. And what of the financial outlay? Previously where a stroke victim was assessed and the conclusion reached was that little or no recovery could be expected, recovery of a high level became possible and a long stay in hospital greatly reduced. Probably the greatest factor which has contributed to the belief of many doctors that no adequate recovery of the severely disabled hemiplegic patient is possible springs from their observation over many years that **this has been the case**. It is frustrating to feel that much more education is necessary at the grass roots of medical schools, nursing schools and sometimes therapy training schools.

The long arm inflatable pressure splint, correctly applied and used over a period of 6 years in the unit of the acute hospital described above seemed to supply the following rehabilitation needs.

1. With all-over *even and sustained pressure* it maintained a total inhibiting pattern.
2. It controlled the distribution of muscle tone in the elbow, wrist and fingers, inhibiting flexion spasticity patterns while rehabilitation took place.

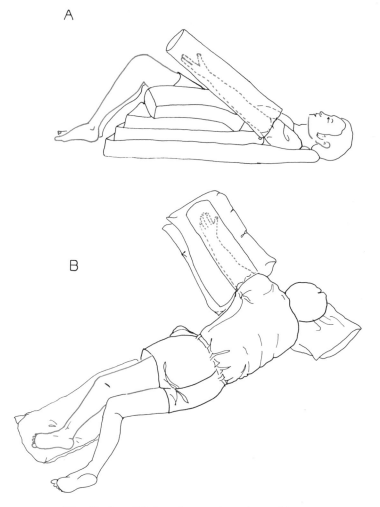

Fig. 17 A and B show therapeutic resting positions.

3. It gave the limb the necessary stability while rehabilitation of the trunk and weightbearing through the shoulder joint were undertaken.

4. It supplied the vital contribution necessary if associated reactions in the hemiplegic arm were to be adequately controlled.

5. It enabled the patient to undertake the constant repetition of exercise necessary for rehabilitation.

6. It was quickly established that it should be used wherever associated reactions or overflow of tone must be directed away from the strong anti-gravity tonal patterns into the opposing weak patterns. Therefore, in my

acute unit, nurses were taught to use it wherever necessary during nursing procedures and during the weekends.

7. It left the therapist's hands free to work with the patient during exercise routines, e.g. to give pain free passive manipulations to maintain a fully mobile wrist or to disturb the patient's balance during balance training.

8. By assisting and making possible the urgent need for early weightbearing through the inhibited wrist and elbow to the inhibited shoulder (the shoulder inhibited *provided* it is maintained and used in outward rotation) it also stimulated joint proprioceptors.

THE LONG ARM SPLINT

Application

This splint is most easily applied with the patient in lying in the total spasticity inhibiting pattern with head extended and rotated towards the affected side, the head position assisting the corrective pattern in the forearm. The splint is applied in three easy stages.

1. The zip fastener is closed, the therapist puts the splint on her own arm (her left arm if it is the patient's left arm, right if it is his right), clasps the patient's hand and draws the patient's arm into the splint, ensuring that his shoulder is outwardly rotated with his elbow, wrist and fingers extended and his thumb abducted.

2. The zip fastener must be on the same side as the patient's little finger *with his fingertips well back from the open end of the splint.*

3. The splint is then fully inflated *by mouth.*

Study Figure 18, which gives a clear step by step diagram of the necessary handholds used to obtain a good resulting full inhibitory pattern. In any situation where it is not easy or suitable to have the patient in lying, the splint may be applied with the patient in a sitting position but try to see that his head is not flexed forward. His head should be held up with neck extension and rotation towards the affected side.

After a trial of all the arm splints that were being marketed (and usually named first aid splints) I found a firm in Denmark who seemed to be using a unique plastic material which answered my purposes and did not become brittle in cold weather. Also the firm in Denmark were prepared to assist me in further development of a series of splints which would deal with the inhibitory and sensory problems faced in stroke rehabilitation. So, it was to Denmark I went.

Remembering that recovery patterns are rotational patterns, outward rotation for the arm, inward rotation for the leg and bilateral rotation for the trunk, trunk rolling is taught early in the rehabilitation programme. Be-

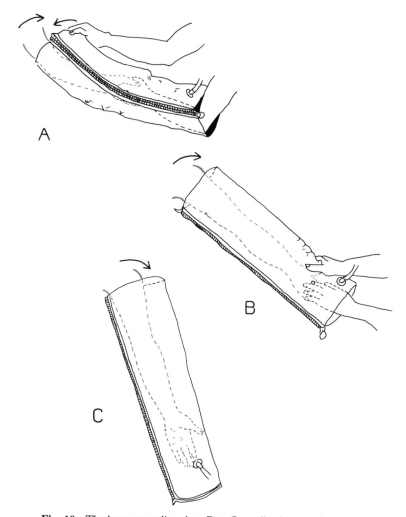

Fig. 18 The long arm splint. A to B to C, application step by step.

cause recovery patterns are usually flexion patterns (except for the forearm and hand) and rolling patterns are flexion patterns, there was a need to protect the vulnerable elbow, wrist and fingers during rolling routines. The simple method of teaching the patient to clasp his hands and reach forward during exercise was not very satisfactory. It was all too easy to bring in an unwanted flexor response in the forearm. Rolling from side to side wearing the long arm splint with both arms stretched forward to shoulder level and knees flexed, was now taught with no fear of stepping up unwanted flexor tone in the forearm. The splinted arm was supported by the sound arm. But, where it was necessary to teach a patient to roll over and over across a wide area of floor to stimulate righting reactions (head righting and rotating within the body axis) there seemed a danger of straining the shoulder if the long arm splint was used. Also, to work the upper trunk and to weightbear through the shoulder would only take place where the patient could roll to support himself prone, leaning equally on both elbows and forearms, forearms pointing straight forward to maintain the correct shoulder pattern. In a logical treatment sequence it was necessary to produce a shorter splint to be fitted below the elbow to continue inhibition of wrist and fingers. This led to the development of the half-arm splint. With the splint on, the patient was taught to roll over to prone. He kept both arms stretched forward as before *at shoulder level* so that he completed the roll over evenly supported on both elbows and forearms, with elbows immediately below his shoulders and forearms pointing straight forward. He was stabilised in this position. Now the progression of rolling over and over was undertaken and, with each roll over, he landed correctly in the prone starting position. The correct starting position of every progressive exercise had to be thoroughly stabilised.

THE HALF-ARM SPLINT

Application

It is applied in the same way as the long arm splint but below the elbow, leaving the elbow free for movement. The zip fastener is positioned on the side of the small finger and extends along the ulnar border. It is used:

1. To control tonal distribution in the wrist and fingers as rehabilitation progresses.

2. The patient is able to establish the prone position with forearm propping early in the rehabilitation programme with this splint as an aid. Modification of the starting position may be necessary for the elderly.*

3. By using the prone propping position early in the rehabilitation programme, stability of the head and upper trunk will be established as the therapist leads the patient from assisted work with his head extension to controlled movement and on to resisted movement.

4. By using exercise as in 3, and combining neck extension with rotation towards the affected side, tonic neck reflexes will stimulate the required tonal flow of extension through the forearm.

5. Shoulder stability is established.

6. As described above, the patient may safely undertake the often very necessary progression of rolling over and over across a wide area.

---

* *Restoration of Motor Function in the Stroke Patient.*

THE FOOT SPLINT (see Fig. 19)

This small boot was developed to assist in breaking up the antigravity leg pattern of extension. On trial it was soon seen as an important factor in the prevention of the further development of the abnormal pattern in the already weak ankle and could be invaluable while performing exercises in prone and rolling patterns. It disposed of the need to use pillow support in

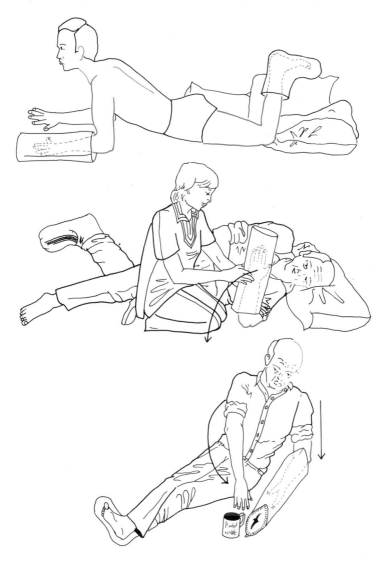

Fig. 19 The half-arm splint in use.

prone lying and also made it possible to weightbear on the point of the heel when in the supine position and in bridging.

Application

The correct application *must* be used. This small boot must be applied with the patient's heel right back into the heel of the splint to give an angle of 90° in the ankle joint. It is applied with the zip open—or closed if you find this easier—and the heel must then be carefully positioned. *Do not* put pressure through the forepart of the sole of the foot as this would bring in an extensor response. With the heel correctly positioned, close the zip (if it is open) and grasp the front of the fabric of the splint to maintain the heel position. As air is blown into the splint gradually release this grasp on the splint. If you cannot apply the boot correctly, *do not use it.* It is used:

1. To assist in maintaining an inhibiting position in the foot while rehabilitation is undertaken.
2. To support the flaccid ankle where necessary or to prevent further development of spasticity but note that this is not a splint for use in standing. If used for weightbearing it will not last very long!

THE HAND SPLINT (see Fig. 20)

This splint was developed to assist in maintaining finger extension and thumb abduction to give a firm weightbearing base in the hand. It is a small double-chamber splint. The splints already developed had only one chamber and consequently only one inflation tube. The hand splint with the two separate compartments (one to cover the back of the hand, and the other to cover the front) has two inflation tubes. Again this is for a sound neurological reason. When applied over the thumb and fingers, with the thumb in abduction with extension and the fingers in extension, if the section which covers the back of the hand is inflated first it will initiate an extensor response in thumb and fingers.

Application

It is applied as described above. The posterior section covering the back of the hand is firmly inflated, then a little air is put into the anterior section to give comfort and a good weightbearing base. Note that this splint is not generally used to control the wrist. It is used:

1. To control thumb and finger positioning, inhibiting flexor spasticity.
2. To assist in establishing weightbearing patterns, for example as in crawling and crawling patterns.

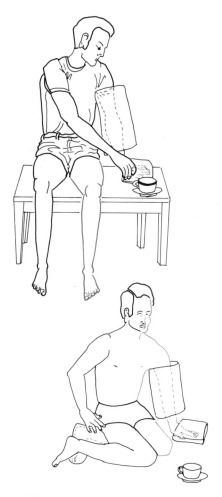

Fig. 20 The hand splint and the elbow splint in use.

3. Stabilising the hand for standing leaning on the hand (see Fig. 21).
4. In any situation where there is a need to inhibit the thumb and fingers.

THE ELBOW SPLINT (see Fig. 20)

This splint was developed to be used in conjunction with the hand splint where the elbow had progressed to a degree of stability but was not yet quite stable enough to support the weightbearing hand in certain exercises. It can be slipped on and off without removing the hand splint if necessary.

Application

It is a short square splint applied with the zip fastener over the anterior aspect of the elbow joint. It should be inflated with the zip fastener close in to the arm to give a large cushion of air over the posterior aspect of the elbow joint.

It is used:

1. To assist in elbow extension.

2. To assist in isolated elbow exercise where weight is transmitted through the hand and elbow flexion and *extension* is obtained by thrusting upward through the positioned hand.

3. As described above, to assist in establishing weightbearing patterns, for example as in crawling and crawling patterns.

THE LEG GAITER (see Fig. 21)

The development of the leg gaiter has proved to be as important to full leg recovery as the long arm splint is to full arm recovery, recovery meaning a

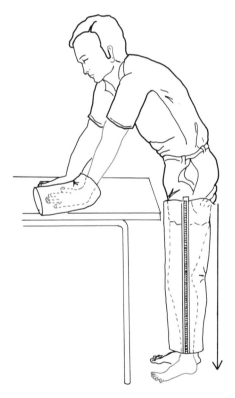

Fig. 21 The leg gaiter and the hand and wrist splint.

return to balanced tone and normal patterns of movement. It is a double-chamber leg splint which may be applied in two distinctly different ways.

Application

Its most common use is in the treatment of the hemiplegic leg and the most usual application (*A*) *must be understood.*

A

To apply the splint correctly the patient must be standing comfortably with good arm positioning (splint controlled and weightbearing). His feet should be apart and turned straight forward. The zip fastener on the splint is open and the splint is wrapped round the leg and the zip fastener is then closed. The top edge of the gaiter *must* be high up under the ischial tuberosity and the zip adjusted to ensure that it runs down the centre of the lateral aspect of the leg in line with the trouser seam. This will make sure that the two chambers of the splint are quite clearly placed in anterior and posterior positions.

The posterior chamber is inflated first to a *firm* pressure. As it inflates the patient's weight must be transferred over onto his affected foot. If this is done correctly and his foot is correctly positioned this inflation will bring his affected knee into mild flexion and he will be weightbearing through a correctly positioned hip, thus inhibiting strong extensor antigravity thrust and a consequent build-up of spasticity. Finally, the anterior chamber is inflated minimally to stabilise pressure round the knee. The patient is now ready and able to weightbear through his heel to a semi-flexed knee and a mildly inwardly rotated hip, thus inhibiting the strong action of *Gluteus maximus.*

It is used:

1. For standing training to produce trunk stability using inhibiting limb positioning so that Associated Reactions are fully controlled.

2. For gait training by stepping forwards, backwards and sideways *with the sound leg.* The affected leg remains firmly on the floor in the starting position.

3. For practice in weight transfers from side to side, both feet remaining firmly on the floor. The patient must learn to transfer his weight over to his affected side.

4. For standing practising both knees bending and stretching keeping heels on the floor; this leads to standing on the affected leg only and continuing with the affected knee bending and stretching.

5. All these suggested uses lead to a stable and strong ankle.

Note. This gaiter is not intended as a walking splint.

B

Where the hemiplegic leg goes into flexion and the patient stands only on his sound leg the second method of application of the leg gaiter will be required. This is not a common condition but it does occur occasionally. As far as I know this has not yet been fully explained but I have found it to occur in previously pinned hips or in association with pain in the lumbar region and have thought it may be a withdrawal reflex. If this problem does occur it must be faced with a satisfactory rehabilitation approach and the second method of application of the leg gaiter has supplied this need. As already described, the leg gaiter is wrapped round the leg and the zip fastener is closed. The gaiter is carefully positioned as before but the patient is lying comfortably supported on his back. In this second method of application *the anterior chamber is inflated first* to give firm support with the knee in extension. The posterior chamber is inflated next to give all-round stability to the leg and the patient is assisted into a standing position with both feet in a suitable weightbearing position.

It will be readily understood that this second method of application (*B*) of the leg gaiter *must not be used* on the much more usual tonal pattern of the hemiplegic patient where the need is to inhibit antigravity tone and, in particular, the antigravity leg pattern which is mainly established by the strong action of *Gluteus maximus* where it is essential to use the first method of application (*A*).

Again note that this is not a splint to be used for walking and will be used only to assist in obtaining standing balance. The leg withdrawal problem I have not found to persist over a long period where gaiter training is used and the skill of the physiotherapist must be used to monitor tonal patterns correctly and to continue to follow correct rehabilitation principles by treating what she finds.

In all situations the tonal pattern in the arm must be carefully guarded and the build up by associated reactions of excessive antigravity tone should be prevented wherever necessary by the application of the appropriate pressure splint while work takes place on the trunk and legs.

THE HAND AND WRIST SPLINT (see Fig. 21)

This splint is the latest development in the range of splints for the hemiplegic patient. It has been designed to meet the need of the recovering (but still unstable) wrist and hand. Again it is a two chamber splint and is in every detail a repeat of the hand splint *except for the size*. It is considerably larger than the hand splint. Where it is used with the same method of application described for the hand splint (thumb in extension with abduction and fingers in extension) it also supports the wrist. The inflation of the posterior section over the back of the hand and wrist will initiate an extensor response in thumb, fingers and wrist. As a recent development I am already satisfied after using it in the clinical field for 10 weeks that this splint will shorten the time so often necessary to regain hand control. The larger dimensions of this splint also make it a useful tool to be applied to the very large hand to control the thumb and fingers.

STROKE REHABILITATION PRESSURE SPLINTS (see Fig. 22)

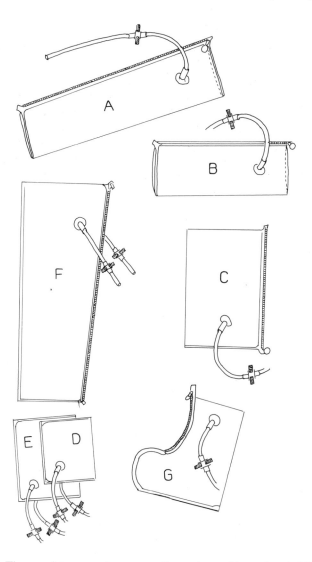

Fig. 22   The complete range of pressure splints to be used in stroke rehabilitation.

A. The long arm splint: available in two sizes: length 70 cm and 80 cm.
B. The half-arm splint: available in one standard size.
C. The elbow splint: available in one standard size.
D. The hand splint: available in one standard size.
E. The hand and wrist splint: available in one standard size.
F. The leg gaiter: available in three sizes: length 60 cm, 70 cm and 75 cm.
G. The foot splint: available in one standard size.

OCCUPATIONAL THERAPY (see Fig. 23)

As this book is intended to meet some of the needs of *all therapists* and, wherever possible, it is hoped that physiotherapists and occupational therapists will be working closely together within a team, Figure 23 is included to illustrate work in an occupational therapy setting. The patient in the diagram is working his upper trunk and shoulder making repetitive movements to reach forward and draw with dots on the white board. Having seen some of the imaginative work produced in this way, and having seen many other examples of the treatment results achieved when physiotherapist and occupational therapist work in perfect harmony, it is to be hoped that this sort of cooperation will have a promising future.

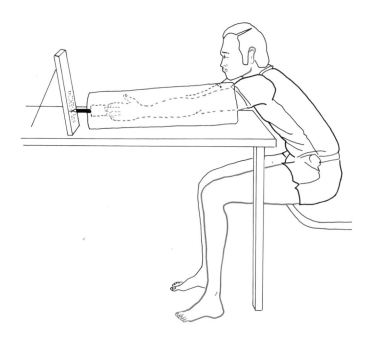

6. Problems

Residual problems found in the stroke patient may be, and frequently are, severe, if treatment is not begun *early* after the onset of the stroke. Preventive treatment for many of these problems occurs quite naturally if correct rehabilitation practices are followed. To understand why some of the problems occur and how to treat potential problems, is to reduce the chance of the development of severe and often intractible disability thus preventing much unnecessary suffering for the patient. For example, the agony shoulder of the stroke patient at once springs to mind. It is not difficult to prevent this unnecessary distress provided the cause is understood.

THE SHOULDER JOINT

Why does the shoulder joint give trouble?

1. Because it is a lax joint at the best of times.
2. Because it is dependent on the normal plane of the joint between scapula and humerus.
3. Because it is dependent on a normal supraspinatus muscle.
4. Because it is dependent on the rotator cuff ligament.
5. Because it is dependent on a mobile scapula.

After a stroke all of these factors may be affected.
Hemiplegic shoulder pain is due to:

1. Altered plane of the joint.
2. Muscle weakness.
3. A lax ligament.
4. An immobile scapula.

This results in:

1. Impinging of bone surfaces between humerus and scapula.
2. Pinching of the rotator cuff.
3. Damage to supraspinatus.

Damage occurs:

1. If the patient is rolled over onto a disabled shoulder which is trapped below his body weight in inward rotation.

2. If the patient is pulled up the bed by an inwardly rotated shoulder.

3. If the patient is assisted in any way by pulling on or weightbearing through an inwardly rotated shoulder.

4. If the patient's upper trunk and shoulder, particularly the scapula, are not therapeutically treated to establish and maintain upper trunk and scapula mobility.

5. If lacking tone is not restored.

Treatment

1. All treatment should be undertaken with the long arm splint in place to divert all overflow of tone into the inhibiting pattern for elbow, wrist and fingers.

2. Mobilise the upper trunk. Remember that *Latissimus dorsi* has extensive origins in the trunk and spasticity of this area may occur fairly rapidly after the stroke giving side flexion with shortening of the trunk and retraction with inward rotation of the shoulder.

3. Keep the scapula mobile so that free movement allows it to slide round the chest wall.

4. Therapists work to mobilise and maintain the necessary outward rotation of the shoulder.

5. Nurses must always use this shoulder pattern of outward rotation in their handling of the patient. Do physiotherapists teach this where necessary? If not, why not? All members of any team, hospital or home based should understand this vital need.

6. Get tone into the shoulder as quickly as possible by giving compression through the outwardly rotated shoulder joint. If it hurts you are doing something wrong. Make sure the shoulder is in outward rotation and there must be firm support behind the scapula.

7. Check the weightbearing base (see Fig. 10) and use the arm in the patterns illustrated in Figure 7, prone, and Figure 9, crawling. Crawling will be a later progression.

8. **Stabilise** the upper trunk and shoulder while using the prone position (Fig. 7).

9. Between physiotherapy sessions supply a shoulder support where it is felt to be necessary but make sure it truly maintains the vital outward rotation. A broad crêpe bandage applied in a figure-of-eight with the cross over at the back and going under alternate axillae but holding a firm supporting pad under the affected shoulder can give very satisfactory support (if correctly applied). If the patient has no objection the bandage may be ap-

plied on the top of clothing where it is seen as a reminder to all helpers that the shoulder must be handled with great care.

SUBLUXATION OF THE SHOULDER

Subluxation of the shoulder will be found in many weak stroke shoulders but this should not be a problem provided it is handled as suggested above. Subluxation will not in itself give pain, but, badly handled, it is wide open to receive the injuries listed above. So, take avoiding action and make sure that none of the bad handling which produces damage to the shoulder joint is allowed to take place.

The use of pressure splints and pressure techniques will go a long way towards solving the problems that may have to be faced in stroke rehabilitation and listed below are the suggested solutions that I have found to work.

1. Subluxation of the shoulder

This should not be a problem.

(a) Use a long arm pressure splint and give compression with the shoulder joint in outward rotation.

(b) Give weightbearing in sitting as in Figure 8.

(c) Stabilise also as illustrated in Figure 8.

(d) Use the prone position as in Figure 7 using the half-arm splint. Modify the position if necessary, for example put pillow support under the abdomen or have the patient sitting leaning forward to support himself with parallel forearms on a low table. Stabilise upper trunk and shoulder.

(e) Note that if it hurts you are doing something wrong.

(f) Always check the shoulder position. This means **stay in outward rotation**.

All suggestions are aimed at getting tone into the shoulder.

2. The stiff, painful shoulder

The physiotherapist may inherit this problem when she takes over a patient for late treatment.

(a) There is usually spasticity in the trunk.

(b) Start with the trunk but first apply a long arm splint.

(c) Position the patient lying on his sound side as in Figure 17B but have him lying over a pillow to elongate the trunk. Start with a rest period in this position.

(d) Same position: separately teach upper and lower trunk rotations.

Start with passive mobilisation, progress to active assisted work and then on to active work.

(e)   Same position: manually mobilise the scapula with one hand while supporting the splinted arm with the other hand. Deep frictions round the posterior scapula border will be useful and a comfortable oil massage to the whole area.

(f)   Same position: trunk rolling in opposite rotations.

(g)   Roll the patient onto his back with his legs in the crook position, support the splinted arm in elevation with outward rotation and mobilise the shoulder using your free hand to support the scapula and to assist in mobilising the shoulder in protraction.

(h)   Roll back into the side-lying position and mobilise the shoulder by assisting the splinted arm in a sawing movement across the pillow which is supporting the arm.

Long term flaccidity (or hypotonicity)

Probably the most difficult problem of all.

(a)   Apply a full arm splint.

(b)   To increase tone use weightbearing patterns.

(c)   There is usually a need to substantially increase sensory input.

(d)   Add two daily sessions of at least one hour each of intermittent pressure to stimulate muscular proprioceptors.

(e)   Use compression techniques to stimulate joint proprioceptors.

(f)   Where available the tilt table can be used to great advantage, with arm weightbearing included, making prolonged weightbearing possible.

(g)   Lying prone on positioned forearms as in Figure 7 with the half-arm splint in position and using the sound arm in various movements to distribute weight through the affected arm.

(h)   Remember that flexor spasticity may develop even in the formerly flaccid arm *if* inhibiting patterns are not carefully maintained at all times. Carefully assess your progress.

(i)   Use tapping and pounding. Also *quick* ice treatment may have a place here.

This sort of treatment will often give very satisfactory results.

The inverted spastic foot

This is frequently the result of lack of the correct early care. It is not a problem where rocking chair and gaiter training for the leg are used in early rehabilitation.

Late treatment:

(a) If possible manually stretch the Achilles Tendon but do not do this by applying pressure to the forepart of the foot. That would simply increase the spasticity.

(b) Go back to the beginning and check recovery in the lower trunk and hip. Any weakness or spasticity in this area must be dealt with.

(c) As suggested above, use the rocking chair with careful positioning of the hip and foot.

(d) Use weightbearing in inhibiting position—study the correct foot position as illustrated in Figure 10 and apply the leg gaiter correctly. Then follow the given exercises, particularly number 4 on page 69. In all the gaiter exercises keep the heel firmly on the floor.

(e) In mat work, bridging is useful but inhibit strongly over the foot; this should be achieved by the physiotherapist bending up the toes, particularly the great toe, with weightbearing through the point of the heel.

(f) Use sitting to standing from a low stool with the affected foot carefully positioned. Remember in sitting to standing the sound foot should be just in front of the affected foot, the foot in front taking less weight than the foot behind. Use the long arm splint to take care of associated reactions.

(g) Do not use a rigid foot splint; use a lively splint if any. I would recommend the Air-stirrup Ankle Training Brace as marketed by Aircast, if any. But it is no use to tackle the problem from the wrong end. This means that full recovery will only take place if it comes from the hip downwards. See (b) above. However, the anti-spasticity pattern of the total leg must be maintained at all times and carefully used for all exercise routines, particularly for weightbearing, with the ankle protected against increasing spasticity and undue strain while recovery takes place from above downwards. I have found (d) above of particular value in this situation.

Oedema of the hand

This is not a problem where pressure techniques are used, but, if it occurs, as may be the case where late treatment is offered, it should be dealt with promptly.

(a) Use pressure splints for treatment sessions and give passive manipulations with the full arm splint inhibiting the spasticity pattern (even if the arm is flaccid). For example, give wrist extension and flexion.

(b) Use positioning at all times and include positioning with elevation where necessary.

(c) Include sessions of treatment with intermittent pressure, provided there are no contra-indications. Contra-indications for any use of intermittent pressure in stroke care: it should not be used on patients in acute pulmonary oedema and should be used with caution on those with congestive heart failure or in those where pre-existing deep veinous thrombosis is suspected. For the severely oedematous hand use intermittent pressure with limb elevation.

(d) Inhibiting positioning where the arm is not allowed to hang down from the shoulder is particularly important.

(e) Use weightbearing exercise with long arm pressure splint support in inhibiting patterns.

(f) Constantly remind the patient to position his own arm—the golden rule: *Wherever possible hand over the care of his own limbs to the patient himself.*

(g) It is necessary to supply a suitable arm rest, for example a gutter arm rest on the chair. This is a necessity for all arm rehabilitation so that the patient may safely sit in an inhibiting arm pattern.

Loss of the memory of movement

In the days immediately following a stroke the patient's brain will readily forget established movement patterns and will readily adopt new, abnormal patterns. This can quickly establish a major barrier to successful rehabilitation as it is enormously difficult to reverse abnormal patterns and restore normal patterns. Loss of kinaesthetic memory is a negative sign. Man can only do movements which he has experienced before. There seems to be a complete wiping out of memory and it is useless to expect to do movement with the sound side and imitate with the affected side. The brain will not connect the two. The patient must relearn the feeling of movement—no wonder sensory loss can present such a rehabilitation problem. The case for stepping up sensory input has been given; now the patient needs repetition, over and over again in movement patterns and in exercise patterns but these must be done with sustained pressure maintaining inhibiting patterns. For the realisation of a movement you have to make it possible. The patient is bound to coordinate wrong movement unless he has the memory of correct movement. Treatment consists of making him able to remember the normal movement. He may be in an endless vicious circle, a vicious circle of abnormal input and output, he may even be paralysed, and treatment must break this vicious circle. Treatment should be early before this becomes a major problem. *Step up sensory input before this becomes a major problem and give repetition over and over again.* But this must be the rule for all stroke rehabilitation with emphasis on the need to *start treatment early.*

Summary

(a) There are positive and negative signs. *Positive* = too much movement and the patient overshoots his target. *Negative* = loss of function.

(b) The brain forgets established movement patterns.

(c) The brain quickly adopts new abnormal patterns.

(d) This quickly establishes a major barrier to rehabilitation.

(e) Loss of kinesthetic memory seems to be a complete wiping out of memory.

(f) No use to expect to do movement with sound side and mimic with affected side. Brain will not connect the two.

(g) **Treatment** must be early, stepping up sensory input and giving repetition over and over again with passive and inhibitory controlled movement patterns.

(h) Attempt to get the patient's full concentration and ask him to 'think the movement' as you perform it passively. Attempt to get his memory to retain the normal pattern and gradually let him take over, going through the stages of active assisted movement to active movement.

(i) A quiet room will be necessary for this kind of treatment.

(j) Again it is essential to base the rehabilitation programme on neurodevelopmental patterns.

I find that loss of the memory of movement is much less of a problem since I started to use pressure techniques with inhibiting patterns and increased sensory input. The whole concept of treatment rests with the need to restore *normal postural tone* and a normal postural reflex mechanism. Note that walking, for example, is a constant process of losing and regaining balance.

Extensor spasticity in the leg

This will often be found if early and correct practices in rehabilitation have not been established early after the onset of the stroke. However, once again with the intervention of pressure splint techniques, reversing this abnormal tonal pattern is possible. Rehabilitation stages should be understood.

(a) Teach and use inhibiting positioning at all times.

(b) Give passive movements in inhibiting patterns but the position of the physiotherapist's hands is of extreme importance. For example, she must not place a hand under the forepart of the foot to assist hip and knee flexion—this will only assist the thrust downwards into extension. The hand should be placed firmly under the heel while the operator's second hand will direct the movement into inward rotation with flexion of the hip.

(c) Change passive movements into assisted active movements as rehabilitation advances, and work towards unassisted voluntary movement.

(d) Use placing and movement in inhibiting patterns.

(e) Use leg gaiter training as already described to encourage weightbearing through the heel of a correctly positioned foot, distributing weight up through a semi-flexed knee to an inwardly rotated hip. This will inhibit the strong thrust of *Gluteus maximus* and increase tone in the low tonal pattern of flexion.

(f)   Follow through the leg gaiter exercise progressions as already given in Chapter 5, application of the leg gaiter, Method *A*.

(g)   The use of the rocking chair,* provided careful inhibiting positioning is used, will be much more beneficial than the use of a static chair. With careful foot positioning the patient will use his leg within an inhibiting pattern with each rock of the chair. Positioning (as in all instances) must include arm positioning.

Note. A footboard for bed rest must never be used. If a footboard is used, the front part of the patient's foot will push against it, bringing in an extensor response and increasing the unwanted extensor spasticity.

The pusher syndrome

The pusher syndrome, or the persistent lateral lean, presents a situation which many find difficult to treat successfully. However, far from it being a severe complication which interferes with satisfactory rehabilitation, it can be used to give positive assistance in the treatment programme.

The average stroke patient cannot and will not transfer his weight across to the affected side of his body. He will move from sitting to standing, compensating for his loss of function by using his sound side. This means that he stands up taking all his weight only on his unaffected side, using his hemiplegic leg as no more than a prop, toes in contact with the ground, and antigravity tone will usually develop at an alarming rate giving the all too familiar picture of spasticity as described above. As recovery depends on re-establishing a balanced body with normal muscle tone, it is essential that he should aim to recover normal standing balance. To do this his advancing rehabilitation programme must use weightbearing through both sides of his body with inhibiting positions guarding against the onset (and ever increasing problem) of spasticity. As the whole concept of treatment rests with the need to restore normal postural tone, the patient must be taught to transfer his weight over onto his affected side and then progress to trunk stability with even tonal distribution through both sides of body. It sometimes takes many weeks of training before the patient is able to stand with sound standing balance.

The patient with the pusher syndrome presents with a totally opposite situation. Here, when the patient attempts to stand, he pushes strongly through his sound leg to stand up and, as he stands, all his weight is thrown

---

*   Refer to *Restoration of Motor Function in the Stroke Patient*, Margaret Johnstone, Churchill Livingstone, 1987, Third Edition.

across to his affected side in a dangerous lateral lean which his hemiplegic side cannot support. Even if he is fully supported on his affected side by a helper, she will not be able to cope with the demand made on her, particularly where the overweight patient is concerned. They may both finish on the floor. The pusher syndrome is usually a sign of severe sensory loss.

This apparently disastrous situation described as the pusher syndrome will be best turned to the patient's advantage in the following treatment sequence:

(a) Early daily training in rolling is essential and should lead as soon as possible into rolling over and over (rotating within the body axis) right across a large floor space. For this routine the patient's hands will be clasped and held up above his head.

(b) Mat work to include all head and neck routines and trunk stabilising with stability given to the hemiplegic arm by a long arm pressure splint.

(c) Daily training in standing balance should also start early. The Arjo Lift Walker presently found in many physiotherapy departments gives ideal patient support but it may also require two therapists to help the patient into standing, suitably positioned, and then to *apply two gaiters*, one to each leg. The gaiters must be positioned high up under the ischial tuberosities and applied as given for Method *A* in Chapter 5. The hemiplegic arm should also be carefully positioned in ulnar border leaning if possible. This is easily achieved where there is an Arjo Lift Walker available. The half-arm splint is used and both arms are positioned leaning on parallel forearms.

(d) With the whole of the hemiplegic side of the body well supported with the help of pressure splints the patient is now fully weightbearing *through his affected side* which is positioned in inhibiting patterns. Without the pusher syndrome this is often very slow to be established. With the pusher syndrome it is quickly and easily established provided both legs are supported by leg gaiters and the pelvis is balanced.

(e) Trunk stabilising techniques are used with the patient positioned as in (d). Note that it is also essential to continue the daily sessions in rolling.

So, is the pusher syndrome a rehabilitation bonus? I believe it can be because the essential early training using techniques which demand the ability to weightbear in inhibiting patterns through the affected side of the body are very quickly established. Rolling and weightbearing will stimulate proprioceptors and dynamic trunk stabilising techniques are undertaken at a very early stage in rehabilitation. It will be necessary to train the patient to transfer his weight over to his sound side before a fully balanced trunk is finally achieved, but take advantage of the time when he cannot transfer weight to his sound side and give all the weightbearing techniques that demand full weight through inhibited hemiplegic limbs and successful results are often excellent.

Where the hemiplegic leg goes into flexion and the patient stands only on his sound leg (which is not a common occurrence but it does sometimes happen) refer to the section on splints (Ch. 5) and application of the leg gaiter Method *B*.

Control of associated reactions

Physiotherapists may use different terminology; they may think in different ways and will refer to:

(a) Associated reactions.
(b) Overflow of tone.
(c) Irradiation.

But all should be thinking of the total tonal patterns that will occur with all movement and, in particular, of the alteration of tonal patterns that will occur in the hemiplegic side of the patient's body with every movement made with his sound side because of abnormal reflex activity. For example: *never give the patient a walking stick* to use on his sound side. To do this is to destroy rehabilitation progress. He will simply learn to lean on the stick and to substitute lost function in his affected side by compensating with his sound side. From then on treatment progress will stop because he is now steadily producing non-inhibited antigravity tonal patterns on his affected side. *If you are not going to inhibit 24 hours a day, why bother to treat at all.*

Note that pressure splints are not used for 24 hours a day. They are used for treatment sessions to make it possible to obtain limb stability and to perform the exercises in inhibiting patterns which recovery demands. The long arm splint may be left on for a full hour for resting periods and to precede an exercise session but it should not be left on at night. Between periods of splint use make it possible for the patient to rest in inhibiting patterns by using the necessary supporting furniture.*

To control associated reactions:

(a) Maintain inhibiting patterns.
(b) Make tonal overflow work for you and not against you.
(c) Direct this overflow into *the low tonal patterns*.
(d) Where necessary use pressure splint support.

Gross sensory loss

Where there is loss of proprioceptive sense it is essential to add intermittent pressure to the treatment programme to give movement within the tissues.

---

* Refer to *Home Care for the Stroke Patient*, Margaret Johnstone, Churchill Livingstone, 1987, Second Edition.

(Sensory nerves accommodate to sustained pressure.) There are various pumps on the market but the machine which I have tried and tested for the longest period of time is the British Flowpulse 1100 machine. This machine offers:

Pressure: Variable 20–100 mmHg.
Inflation time: Variable in steps 3 seconds–4 minutes.
Deflation time: Variable in steps 3 seconds–4 minutes.
Treatment time: Variable up to 1 hour.

I have used this pressure pump with different timing for two different purposes:
1. Where there is sensory loss
   (a) Pressure 1 : 40 mmHg . . . . for 3 seconds
   (b) Pressure 2 : 10 mmHg . . . . for 3 seconds
                                              Time 45 minutes

Treatment was given twice daily.

2. To treat oedema
   (a) Pressure 1 : 40 mmHg . . . . for 10 seconds
   (b) Pressure 2 : 10 mmHg . . . . for 15 seconds
                                            Time 1–1¹/₂ hours.

Treatment was given twice daily.

Conclusion

The sensorimotor approach to stroke rehabilitation as described here is a reasoned and satisfying approach which gives consistently good results. With a breakdown in the finely balanced facilitatory–inhibitory principle on which the neuromuscular system depends, therapists and all who care for stroke patients must act as an extended facilitatory–inhibitory agent until normal responses are re-established and cortical control regained.

This means that all should understand the inhibiting positions that must be used at all times until cortical control is regained. If we fail in this basic need is it the fault of the physiotherapist? Is it a failure to communicate with families? Are physiotherapists in the right place or should there be more of them in the home and less of them in hospitals? Are there enough to go round? These are questions that still need to be solved.

7. Case history to illustrate the use of pressure techniques

The photographs that follow (Figs 24–38) show advancing rehabilitation with URIAS pressure splint support. This may be described as an air support system used to stabilise and maintain limbs in inhibiting patterns while a reasoned and neurologically sound rehabilitation programme is undertaken. It is now called the Johnstone Concept. Carefully implemented and now used in various parts of the world it is giving very satisfactory results. It should be understood that the young man presented in the photographs had had 12 months of careful hospital therapy *before* the course of treatment with pressure techniques was started. The photographs, therefore, show treatment beginning 1 year *after* the onset of a subarachnoid haemorrhage. At this time, 1 year after onset, he was discharged from hospital rehabilitation with the following disabilities:

1. Marked hemiplegic gait—left-sided.
2. Spasticity of trunk, leg and arm, most severe in the arm—left-sided.
3. Various sensory loss including proprioceptive loss as tests showed loss of proprioceptive sense in elbow and hand, also in his foot but less marked here. His geometric drawings were poor. For mental capacity he scored 10 out of 10.
4. As might be expected, he presented with wrist flexion and a tightly fisted hand on an inwardly rotated and useless arm.

At this stage he was told that rehabilitation could do no more for him. One of the basic rules for satisfactory return of function is that treatment must start *early* after onset of a CVA—the author considers this rule to be vital to optimum recovery. To accept such residual and severe disability (perhaps particularly in a *young* man) seems a very wrong practice. But, to reverse such severe disability *is not an easy task* and is quite impossible without the use of pressure techniques and intensive treatment which usually requires a family commitment.

The photographs and the test chart of gross motor performance which is included after the photographs show the progress made over a 15-month period *after* discharge from hospital rehabilitation. An unfinished rehabilitation is presented as the young man is presently in the middle of this course of treatment and the photographs give a fair representation of some of the pressure techniques that are currently in use. There is no reason to suppose that full rehabilitation will not be achieved. Hand recovery has now begun and is following the same satisfactory sequence which has been demonstrated in many other patients who have regained voluntary responses and learned skills (full cortical control).

Figures 24–38

Note. The date of onset of the subarachnoid haemorrhage was August 1988.

The start of the pressure techniques and of the photographs was approximately 1 year later.

Treatment venue. Treatment took place in the client's home with his father's support and physiotherapy supervision.

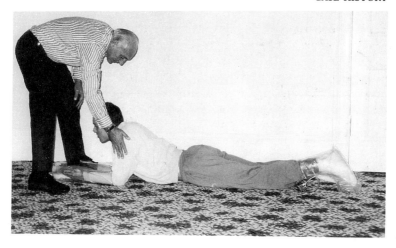

Fig. 24 *Half-arm splint* and *foot splint*: stabilising the upper trunk and shoulder with family involvement—father assists his son.

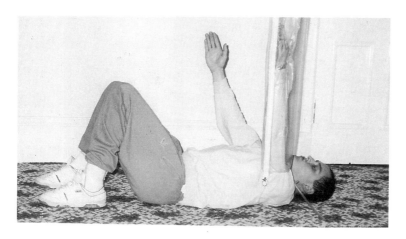

Fig. 25 *Long arm splint*: a 'placing' response has now been obtained.

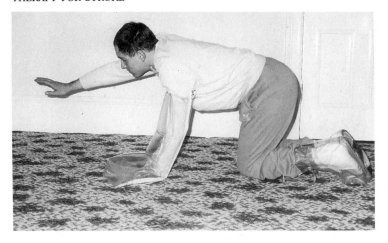

Fig. 26 *Long arm splint* and *foot splint*: attempting to establish the crawling position with transfer of weight through the affected side—but not enough outward rotation of the arm.

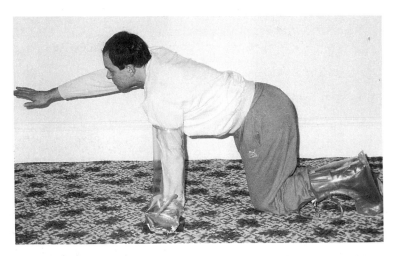

Fig. 27 As in Figure 26 but note the outward rotation of the affected arm and the improved thrust through the arm.

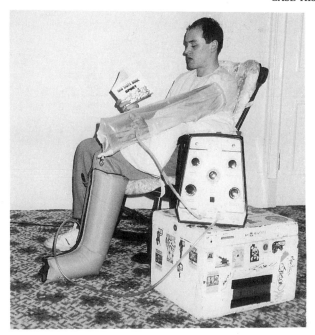

Fig. 28 Intermittent pressure for sensory loss.
Pressures 40 mmHg for 3 seconds
10 mmHg for 3 seconds } for 1 hour twice daily.

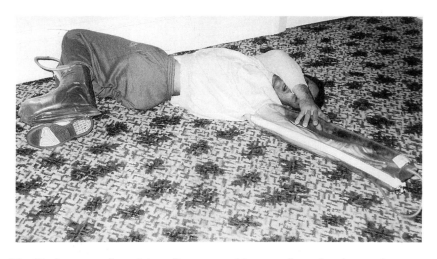

Fig. 29 *Long arm splint* and *foot splint*: upper and lower trunk rotations in opposite directions.

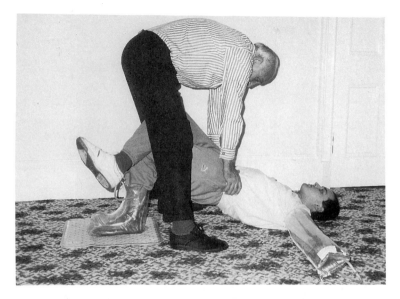

Fig. 30   *Long arm splint* controls tonal flow into the affected arm.

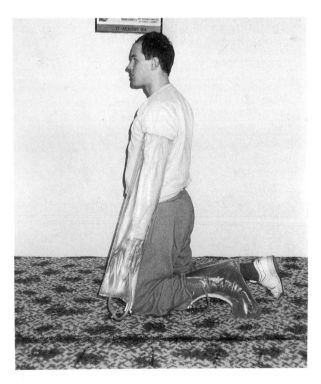

Fig. 31   High kneeling balance established. Knee walking with inhibiting arm and foot pattern maintained by splint stability.

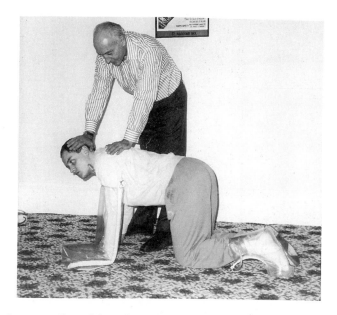

Fig. 32 *Long arm splint* and *foot splint*: stabilising and controlling tonal flow while reinforcing thrust through the inhibited arm.

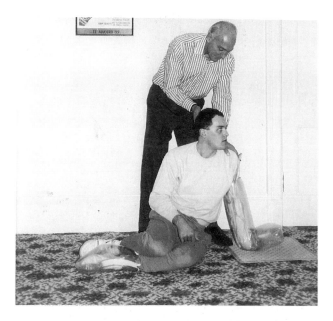

Fig. 33 Stabilising in a good sitting position.

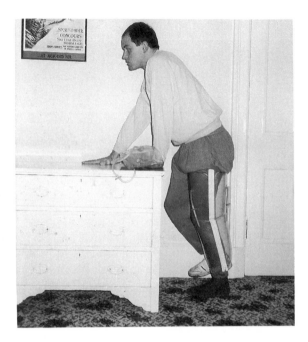

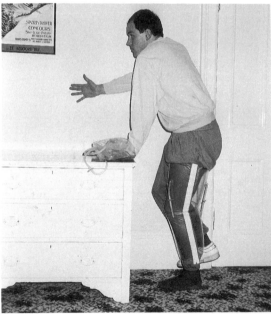

Fig. 34 *Leg gaiter* and *hand splint*: practising weightbearing through the affected side of his body using splint-supported inhibiting patterns.

Note. When applying the leg gaiter, inflating the posterior section will maintain the necessary inhibiting position of mild knee flexion with the heel firmly on the ground. This will only happen if the foot is correctly positioned and weight is transferred over the foot as inflation takes place.

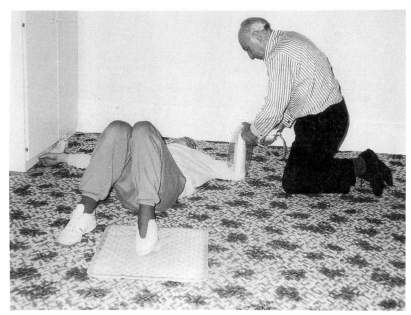

A

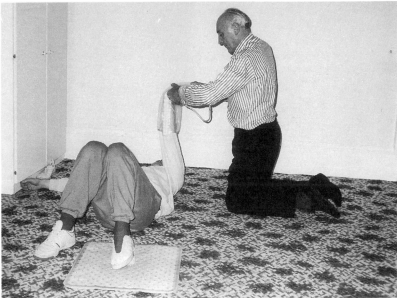

B

Fig. 35 *Half arm splint*: wrist held in extension, thrusting the arm upward against carefully graduated resistance.
A = starting position, B = finishing position.
  Note. Rehabilitation of the upper trunk and shoulder is completed, including strong shoulder protraction. Elbow recovery is well advanced **but** the improved arm function must be maintained as rehabilitation advances to the lower arm, wrist and fingers.

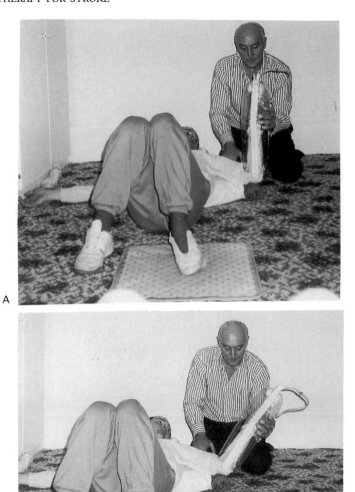

Fig. 36 *Half-arm splint*: retraining isolated elbow movement into extension. A = starting position, B = mid-position and C = finishing position.

Note. Loss of kinaesthetic memory, or loss of the memory of normal movement, can give problems and this can be particularly true of elbow extension using triceps.

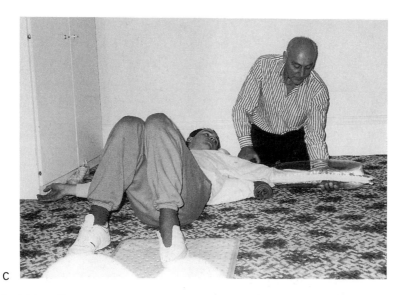

C

Fig. 36 (contd)

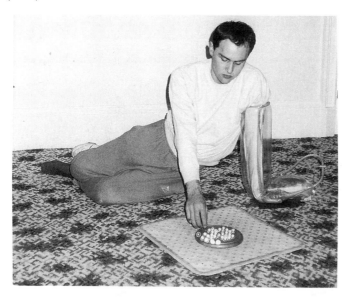

Fig. 37 *Full arm splint*: demonstrating a useful sitting position in which to carry out a task. (An example of 'living in a recovery pattern'.)

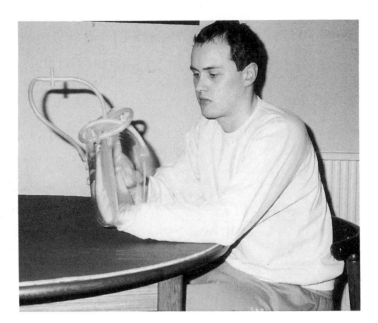

Fig. 38   *The hand splint* is used here in self-care retraining of wrist extension. (Criticism: teach him to place his forearm more firmly on the table so that there is total forearm and *elbow* support.)

Note. When applying the splint, inflate the posterior section first to bring in an extensor response in the fingers.

NAME   Age   24
DIAGNOSIS   R Cerebral artery haemorrhage   Occupation   Student
DATE OF ONSET August 1988
DATE OF START   of pressure techniques
                        one year after onset
TREATMENT VENUE in his own home with family support

CHART OF GROSS MOTOR PERFORMANCE one year after CVA (see dates above)

Scale of grading:- 3 = unaided, 2 = with minimal help, 1 = with help,
                            0 = impossible.

GROSS MOTOR PERFORMANCE: IN BED

DATE	2/8/89	5/10/89	11/1/90	20/6/90	19/10/90
1. Roll from supine to right	3	3	3	3	3
2. Roll from supine to left	3	3	3	3	3
3. Bridging	1+	2	3	3	3
4. Roll to elbow propping	1+	2	3	3	3
5. Roll to sitting over edge of bed	2	2	3	3	3
6. Sitting without use of hands	2	2+	3	3	3
7. Transfer from bed to chair	3	3	3	3	3

GROSS MOTOR PERFORMANCE: IN PHYSIO.

1. Rolling to prone lying	2+	3	3	3	3
2. Prone lying with forearm support	1+	2	2+	3	3
3. Kneeling with forearm support	2	2	2+	3	3
4. Full kneeling to stand kneeling	2	2	3	3	3
5. Crawling	0	1	2	2	2+

GROSS MOTOR PERFORMANCE: BALANCE

1. In sitting	3	3	3	3	3
2. In kneeling	2	2+	3	3	3
3. In standing	2	2+	3	3	3

Fig. 39

GROSS MOTOR PERFORMANCE: WEIGHT TRANSFERS

1. Over affected hip in sitting	②	⑵₊	3	3	3
2. Over affected hand in sitting	⓪	⑴₊	②	⑵₊	⑵₊
3. Cross R leg over L in sitting	3	3	3	3	3
4. Cross L leg over R in sitting	⑴₊	②	⑵₊	3	3
5. Sitting to standing with hands clasped	②	3	3	3	3
6. Over affected hip in standing	②	②	⑵₊	⑵₊	3

Fig. 39 (contd)

Glossary

Agonists	Muscles which contract to produce movement (prime movers) against the weaker antagonists.
Anosognosia	Neglect or denial of ownership of limbs.
Antagonists	Muscles that relax to allow the agonists, or prime movers, to perform a movement.
Approximate	To close together with pressure as used when compression is applied through the articulating surface of a joint.
Apraxia	A disturbance of visual-spatial relationships, or visual-spatial orientation, which leads to inability to deal effectively with or manipulate objects.
Assessment	Informal but careful observation leading to a decision on the state of the patient and the line of treatment to be followed.
Associated reactions	These occur with all attempted movement and are released postural reactions deprived of voluntary control because of cortical damage. They give a widespread increase of spasticity in the affected muscles if the limbs are not inhibited.
Autogenous	Originating within the body.
Body image	The image in an individual's mind of his own body.
Cognition	Knowing or awareness, in the widest sense, including sensation, perception etc. *Awareness*: one of the three aspects of the mind, the others being *affection* (feeling or emotion), and *conation* (willing or desiring). They work as a whole but with cognitive disturbance one may dominate.
Cross facilitation	Working with the sound side of the body across the midline to the affected side to initiate bilateral activity.
Dysarthria	A disorder of speech which includes difficulty in articulation due to motor defect in the muscles of lips, tongue, palate and throat.

99

Dysgraphia	Difficulty in writing.
Dysphasia	A disorder of language which may, or may not, include difficulty in comprehension. More usually comprehension remains intact.
Equilibrium	*Balance*: state of even balance: a state in which opposing forces or tendencies neutralise each other.
Equilibrium responses	See Chapter 3 on reflex activity.
Golgi tendon organs	These are proprioceptors which lie at musculotendinous junctions. They are receptive to sustained stretch and are known to have an inhibitory influence on motoneurone pools of their own muscle supply—an autogenic effect.
Hemianopia	Blindness in one half of the visual field of one or both eyes.
Hypertonia	Excessive or more than normal tone.
Hypotonia	A lack of, or less than normal tone.
Irradiation	Muscle activity which takes place when a strong muscle group acts against resistance to give an overflow of activity (or irradiation) into other parts of the body.
Kinaesthesis	Sense of movement or of muscular effort: perception of movement; kinaesthetic, *adj.*
Neurone	The structural unit of the nervous system comprising fibres (dendrites) which carry impulses to the nerve cell; the nerve itself, and the fibres (axons) which carry impulses from the cell. In the lower motor neurone, the cell is in the spinal cord and the axon passes to skeletal muscle. In the upper motor neurone, the cell is in the cerebral cortex and the axon passes down the spinal cord to arborise with a lower motor neurone.
Parietal lobe	The lobe of the brain which contains the sensory area.
Perception	Act or power of perceiving: discernment: apprehension of any modification of consciousness: the combining of sensations into recognition of an object.
Perseveration	Meaningless repetition of an utterance (or an action as in drawing): tendency to experience difficulty in leaving one thought for another.
Positioning	Placing in the optimum position to allow for, and to promote, recovery.
Prognosis	Forecasting, or forecast, especially in the course of disease.

Proprioceptor	A sensory nerve-ending receptive of sensory stimuli.
Proprioceptive sense	The sense of muscular position, or of muscle and joint position.
P.N.F.	Proprioceptive Neuromuscular Facilitation; methods used to facilitate a response from the neuromuscular mechanism through stimulation of the proprioceptors.
Recovery pattern	The pattern of movement which inhibits dominating reflexes in the stroke patient to allow for, and to promote, recovery. This must also include the resting position, which is the position in which the body is placed to allow for optimum recovery while at rest.
Righting reactions	See Chapter 3 on reflex activity.
Servo mechanism	A mechanism serving automatically to control the working of another mechanism.
Stereognosis	The recognition of familiar objects by their shape, size and texture when held in the hand with the eyes shut.
Synergists	Muscles which contract and relax in conjunction with prime movers crossing more than one joint. *Note.* The synergic pattern of tonic contraction, therefore, results from hypertonic, or excessive, muscle contraction which follows the pattern of the synergists.
Visual agnosia	Failure to interpret what is seen. This type of 'blindness' usually clears up more slowly than hemianopia.

Appendix

Some useful addresses

Aircast
Aircast supply the Air-Stirrup Ankle Brace.
Aircast, PO Box 709, Summit, New Jersey 07902–0709, USA.
In the UK: (Aircast) Orthopaedic Systems, Unit G22, Old Gate, St Michael, Cheshire WA8 8TL (Order = No. 02B/L Single or No. 02B/R Single; write for particulars.)

Arjo
Arjo Lift Walker 214141
Arjo Hospital Equipment is manufactured in Sweden by:
Arjo Hospital Equipment Ltd, Box 61, S–241, Eslöv, Sweden.
Arjo UK Office: Arjo Hospital Equipment Ltd, SPD Building, Acre Road, Reading RG2 OSU.

Medayd Marketing Physiotherapy Suppliers
Useful equipment catalogue available from:
Medayd Marketing Physiotherapy Suppliers, Yew Tree House, 52 Stafford Street, Market Drayton, TF9 1JB.

Flowpulse
Manufactured in Britain: Huntleigh Medical Ltd, Bilton Way, Dallow Road, Luton LU1 1UU.

URIAS
Pressure splints manufactured in Denmark by
Svend Andersen Plastic Industri A/S, DK 4652, Häarlev, Denmark.
UK Agent: Kapitex Healthcare, Kapitex House, 1 Sandbeck Way, Wethersy LS22 4GH.

Index